Male Facial Rejuvenation

Editors

SAMUEL M. LAM
LISA E. ISHII

FACIAL PLASTIC SURGERY CLINICS OF NORTH AMERICA

www.facialplastic.theclinics.com

Consulting Editor
ANTHONY P. SCLAFANI

August 2024 • Volume 32 • Number 3

ELSEVIER

1600 John F. Kennedy Boulevard • Suite 1800 • Philadelphia, Pennsylvania, 19103-2899

http://www.theclinics.com

FACIAL PLASTIC SURGERY CLINICS OF NORTH AMERICA Volume 32, Number 3
August 2024 ISSN 1064-7406, ISBN-13: 978-0-443-13131-8

Editor: Stacy Eastman
Developmental Editor: Malvika Shah

Facial Plastic Surgery Clinics of North America (ISSN 1064-7406) is published quarterly by Elsevier Inc., 360 Park Avenue South, New York, NY 10010-1710. Months of issue are February, May, August, and November. Business and Editorial Offices: 1600 John F. Kennedy Blvd., Suite 1800, Philadelphia, PA 19103-2899. Periodicals postage paid at New York, NY, and additional mailing offices. Subscription prices are $432.00 per year (US individuals), $487.00 per year (Canadian individuals), $579.00 per year (foreign individuals), $100.00 per year (US students), $100.00 per year (Canadian students), and $255.00 per year (foreign students). For institutional access pricing please contact Customer Service via the contact information below. Foreign air speed delivery is included in all *Clinics* subscription prices. All prices are subject to change without notice. POSTMASTER: Send address changes to *Facial Plastic Surgery Clinics*, Elsevier Health Sciences Division, Subscription Customer Service, 3251 Riverport Lane, Maryland Heights, MO 63043. **Customer service: 1-800-654-2452 (US and Canada); 1-314-447-8871 (outside US and Canada); Fax: 314-447-8029; E-mail: journalscustomerservice-usa@elsevier.com (for print support); journalsonline-support-usa@elsevier.com (for online support).**

Reprints. For copies of 100 or more of articles in this publication, please contact the Commercial Reprints Department, Elsevier Inc., 360 Park Avenue South, New York, NY 10010-1710. Tel.: 212-633-3874; Fax: 212-633-3820; E-mail: reprints@elsevier.com.

Facial Plastic Surgery Clinics of North America is covered in *MEDLINE/PubMed* (*Index Medicus*).

Contributors

CONSULTING EDITOR

ANTHONY P. SCLAFANI, MD, MBA, FACS
Director of Facial Plastic Surgery,
Professor of Otolaryngology - Head & Neck
Surgery, Weill Cornell Medical College, New
York, NY

EDITORS

SAMUEL M. LAM, MD, FACS, FISHRS
Director, Willow Bend Wellness Center, Plano,
Texas, USA

LISA E. ISHII, MD, MHS
Senior Vice President, Operations, Johns
Hopkins Health System, Professor,
Otolaryngology–Head and Neck Surgery,
Johns Hopkins University, Baltimore,
Maryland, USA

AUTHORS

PARIS JASMINE AUSTELL, MD, MBA
Facial Plastic and Reconstructive Surgery
Fellow, The Williams Center for Plastic Surgery,
Latham, New York, USA

JASON D. BLOOM, MD, FACS
Facial Plastic and Reconstructive Surgery,
Department of Otolaryngology–Head and Neck
Surgery, University of Pennsylvania,
Philadelphia, Pennsylvania, USA; Facial Plastic
& Reconstructive Surgeon, Bloom Facial
Plastic Surgery, Bryn Mawr, Pennsylvania,
USA

**CRAIG CAMERON BRAWLEY, MD, MS,
MBA**
Clinical Instructor, Department of
Otolaryngology–Head and Neck Surgery,
Division of Facial Plastic and Reconstructive
Surgery, NYU Grossman School of Medicine,
New York City, New York, USA

DOMINIC BRAY, FRCSEd (ORL-HNS)
Facial Plastic Surgeon, Facial Plastic Surgery,
Dominic Bray Facial Plastic Surgery, London,
United Kingdom

EMILY C. DEANE, MD, FRCSC, MSc
Facial Plastic and Reconstructive Surgery
Fellow, Department of Otolaryngology–Head
and Neck Surgery, University of Pennsylvania,
Philadelphia, Pennsylvania, USA

JEFFREY S. EPSTEIN, MD, FACS
Voluntary Assistant Professor, Department of
Otolaryngology, University of Miami, Miami,
Florida, USA

JOHN W. FREDERICK, MD
Facial Plastic Surgeon, Department of Facial
Plastic Surgery, Nassif Plastic Surgery, Beverly
Hills, California, USA

JEFFREY T. GU, MD, MS
Department of Otolaryngology–Head and Neck
Surgery, Oregon Health & Science University,
Portland, Oregon, USA

DANIEL B. HALL, MD
Resident, Department of Otolaryngology–Head
and Neck Surgery, The Ohio State University,
Columbus, Ohio, USA

JAE KIM, MD
Facial Plastic Surgeon, Department of Facial Plastic Surgery, Fairfax, Virginia, USA

LESLIE R. KIM, MD, MPH
Clinical Associate Professor, Department of Otolaryngology–Head and Neck Surgery, The Ohio State University, Columbus, Ohio, USA

DANIEL D. LEE, MD
Plastic Surgeon, Williams Center Plastic Surgery Specialists, Latham, New York, USA

LINDA N. LEE, MD
Department of Otolaryngology, Massachusetts Eye and Ear, Assistant Professor, Department of Otolaryngology, Harvard Medical School, Division of Facial Plastic and Reconstructive Surgery, Massachusetts Eye and Ear, Boston, Massachusetts, USA

MYRIAM LOYO, MD, MCR
Associate Professor, Department of Otolaryngology–Head and Neck Surgery, Oregon Health & Science University, Portland, Oregon, USA

PHILIP MILLER, MD
Clinical Professor, Department of Otolaryngology–Head and Neck Surgery, Division of Facial Plastic and Reconstructive Surgery, NYU Grossman School of Medicine, New York City, New York, USA

MICHAEL SOMENEK, MD
Facial Plastic Surgeon, Somenek+Pittman MD, Advanced Plastic Surgery, Washington, DC, USA

BEN TALEI, MD
Surgeon, Beverly Hills Center for Plastic Surgery, Beverly Hills, California, USA

TOM D. WANG, MD
Professor, Department of Otolaryngology–Head and Neck Surgery, Oregon Health & Science University, Portland, Oregon, USA

IVAN WAYNE, MD
Assistant Professor, Department of Otorhinolaryngology, University of Oklahoma College of Medicine, Facial Plastic Surgeon, W Aesthetics, Oklahoma City, Oklahoma, USA

EDWIN FRANCIS WILLIAMS III, MD
Facial Plastic Surgeon, The Williams Center for Plastic Surgery, Latham, New York, USA

ANNI WONG, MD, MS
Facial Plastic and Reconstructive Surgery, Department of Otolaryngology–Head and Neck Surgery, University of Pennsylvania, Philadelphia, Pennsylvania, USA

ROY XIAO, MD, MS
Resident Physician, Department of Otolaryngology, Massachusetts Eye and Ear, Department of Otolaryngology, Harvard Medical School, Boston, Massachusetts, USA

DONALD B. YOO, MD, FACS
Facial Plastic Surgeon, Department of Facial Plastic Surgery, HALO Beverly Hills Plastic Surgery & MedSpa, Beverly Hills, California, USA

Contents

> In this article, the authors describe their preferred advanced deep-plane techniques and modifications that have universally improved outcomes and durability in both men and women. Performing a proper extended deep-plane facelift and neck lift avoids the need to camouflage scars and stigmata of lifts seen in superficial muscu-loaponeurotic system plication and other techniques. In the author's experience, vertical vector deep-plane surgery is more durable, natural, and less reliant on lipo-filling and volume addition. The subtleties of examination and analysis, surgical technique, clinical outcomes, and gender-specific considerations in the reconstruction of gonial and cervicomental angles, deep planar volumetric reduction, facial volumetric change, limited skin delamination, and revision techniques are discussed.

> Direct neck lift offers an excellent surgical technique for men seeking to rejuvenate the neck and avoid a full rhytidectomy. In this chapter, we provide an overview of direct submentoplasty techniques, as well as clinical pearls to consider in the preoperative, intraoperative, and postoperative periods. Different surgical incisions and resultant scars in the anterior neck are discussed and illustrated with figures. Given the degree of variation of submental fullness with which patients present, it is beneficial to be familiar with several different techniques to address the submental and submandibular areas.

> Many different methods achieve male facial augmentation. Arranged from shorter- to longer-term results, these methods include filler, fat/tissue grafting, fat/tissue transposition, and alloplastic implants. This study solely reviews allografts, which provide the most predictable hard-tissue augmentation. An array of alloplasts will be discussed in this study including chin, cheek, mandibular angle, frontal, and temporal implants. The most common and severe complications will also be explored with preventative and treatment algorithms.

of reparative procedures, key aesthetic steps include proper graft dissection so that one- and two-hair grafts contain a minimal cuff of surrounding skin, acute angulation and appropriate direction of recipient sites using the smallest possible recipient-site blades, and aesthetic design.

FACIAL PLASTIC SURGERY CLINICS OF NORTH AMERICA

THE CLINICS ARE AVAILABLE ONLINE!
Access your subscription at:
www.theclinics.com

Foreword
The Niche Market of Male Facial Plastic Surgery

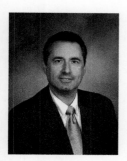

Anthony P. Sclafani, MD, MBA, FACS
Consulting Editor

A man's face is his autobiography. A woman's face is her work of fiction.
> —Oscar Wilde

Wilde's epigram may elicit a wry smile but does point out the traditional social bias that imposes a higher aesthetic standard on women than on men. Women's looks are critiqued and "tweaked"; men are allowed to "mature." Indeed, an overwhelming majority of patients seeking facial plastic surgery in the United States (and even more worldwide) are women. That trend is changing, however, and an increasing number of men are seeking facial plastic surgery, not only for predominantly male issues like male pattern alopecia but also for lines, wrinkles, and sagging skin. Social taboos against men seeking cosmetic care are weakening as society slowly becomes more inclusive, as plastic surgery achieves prominence in the mainstream conversation (in film, news, and especially social media), and as device manufacturers and Big Pharma have recognized the huge untapped market of men. The male patient has distinct aesthetic issues, and surgery should be tailored to these needs as with any patient. Male aesthetic facial plastic surgery has been neglected even as male body surgery has become much more common.

We are beginning to emerge from the fin de siècle attitude skewered in Wilde's quote.

I appreciate the hard work of Drs Lam and Ishii and their esteemed group of authors, and I thank them for sharing their perspectives and expertise in treating the male patient. This issue of *Facial Plastic Surgery Clinics of North America* will enhance your understanding of the unique approaches to, and specific techniques required for, this (potential enormous) minority of facial plastic surgery patients. I am sure you will learn much, to the benefit of your patients. Enjoy!

As I grow older, I pay less attention to what men say. I just watch what they do.
> —Andrew Carnegie

Anthony P. Sclafani, MD, MBA, FACS
Director of Facial Plastic Surgery
Professor of Otolaryngology - Head & Neck Surgery
Weill Cornell Medical College
New York, NY

E-mail address:
ans9243@med.cornell.edu

Facial Plast Surg Clin N Am 32 (2024) ix
https://doi.org/10.1016/j.fsc.2024.03.006
1064-7406/24/

Foreword

The Niche Market of Male Facial Plastic Surgery

Preface
Male Facial Rejuvenation

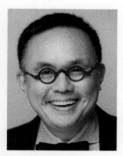

Samuel M. Lam, MD, FACS, FISHRS
Editor

The rise in popularity of facial cosmetic enhancement for men has been spurred on in part by increasing social media awareness. Traditionally, men have been fearful not only of looking unnatural but also for undertaking procedures that they may deem to be uncommon for their gender. However, today with online media celebrating many men revealing their natural transformations, those barriers are quickly falling away. This past year I have performed almost as many facelifts in men as in women. Conversely, I also perform almost as many hair transplants in women as in men, perhaps for similar reasons of stigmas or unawareness for female hair loss diminishing due to online promulgation. I found intriguing the article by Frederick, Yoo, and Kim on Asian male cosmetic surgeries being driven by Korean celebrities–role models of Asian male attractiveness that were absent as I was growing up as an Asian male in the 1980s. The world has become small and fast-paced due to social media along with other societal trends (featured on Netflix, media outlets, and so forth) that have made male cosmetic enhancement now more the norm than taboo. The last issue of *Facial Plastic Surgery Clinics of North America* dedicated to male enhancement was unbelievably in August 2008! Hence, this issue is long overdue. I am proud to have been able to curate and edit this issue with my dear friend and colleague, Lisa Ishii, who has brought her wealth of knowledge and background on the subject as well. I hope that you enjoy and learn as much as I have from the treasure trove of information from these pioneers and thought leaders in our discipline on this burgeoning but in many ways already mature field of surgical and nonsurgical facial cosmetic enhancement for men.

Samuel M. Lam, MD, FACS, FISHRS
Willow Bend Wellness Center
Plano, TX, USA

E-mail address:
drlam@lamfacialplastics.com

Facial Plast Surg Clin N Am 32 (2024) xi
https://doi.org/10.1016/j.fsc.2024.03.007
1064-7406/24/

Preface
A Leap Forward

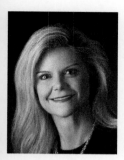

Lisa E. Ishii, MD, MHS
Editor

I am thrilled to share this *Facial Plastic Surgery Clinics of North America* issue focused on male facial rejuvenation. It is a leap forward to devote an entire issue to a heretofore underrepresented focus area. For many years publications focused on methods to restore a more youthful appearance to the aging female face. With this issue we cast a wide net and explore in depth the myriad of options to rejuvenate the male face. From the latest advances in hair transplantation to injectables to implants to surgical approaches tailored to the needs of men, this issue covers the entire spectrum of options. In an era where precision medicine is the goal, this issue provides the latest insights specific to the diverse and fundamental needs of the male patient. Our goal was to compile a comprehensive and practical resource for our colleagues supporting the expanding population of male patients eager to look their best. I thank the readers for allowing us to curate this material on their behalf.

I express my gratitude to the authors of these articles for their expertise in compiling and summarizing the article content. Each author was specifically selected for their reputation and mastery in their niche areas, a fact that will be obvious as the reader immerses themselves in each individual section. The pages spring to life with the energy and enthusiasm the authors hold for their content area, a truly engaging effort. Furthermore, I am grateful to all the authors cited in the individual papers in the references. Without their independent discovery as a foundation, this aggregation of concepts would not be possible.

My coeditor, Dr Sam Lam, is a giant in facial plastic and reconstructive surgery. Dr Lam is a brilliant surgeon and true renaissance man, and partnering with him on this issue was an absolute pleasure. I thank him for his patience and wisdom, and his contagious passion for moving this issue forward.

And finally, I thank my family for their never-ending support and encouragement.

Lisa E. Ishii, MD, MHS
Johns Hopkins Health System
Otolaryngology–Head & Neck Surgery
Johns Hopkins University
733 North Broadway, Suite 105
Baltimore, MD 21287, USA

E-mail address:
Learnes2@jhmi.edu

Facial Plast Surg Clin N Am 32 (2024) xiii
https://doi.org/10.1016/j.fsc.2024.03.008
1064-7406/24/© 2024 Elsevier Inc. All rights reserved.

Male Deep-Plane Face and Neck Lifting
Advanced and Customized Techniques

Dominic Bray, FRCSEd (ORL-HNS)[a],*, Ben Talei, MD[b]

KEYWORDS

- Facelift - Male facelift - Deep-plane facelift - Male neck lift - Deep neck lift - Deep neck reduction
- Deep face contouring

KEY POINTS

- The goals of male facelift patients may differ from those of female patients. Whereas the primary goals for women are youth and beauty, requiring both deep volumetric and superficial skin textural changes, a large proportion of men may seek improvements in the neck and jawline in order to restore masculinity and vigor in addition to youth.
- The word "facelift" in men remains taboo. Primary male facelift candidates will present with concern over loss of neckline definition and will need education and reassurance that necessary extension into the face will not feminize the outcome. Male patients would sooner admit to having a neck lift or blepharoplasty than a facelift, even if all procedures have been performed.
- Most men will judge the success of a facelift by the result in the neck. Without significant improvement in the cervicomental angle and hyoid position, the surgery may be deemed a failure.
- While surgical principles are identical for both sexes, male tissues may be heavier than female soft tissues, requiring a comprehensive deep-plane release to improve results and prevent scarring and failures.
- Specialists performing face and neck surgery should realize that more novel and extensive deep-plane techniques are more widely applicable and are rather uniform between men and women. Certain nuances remain that will improve male outcomes.

INTRODUCTION

Contemporary society has become increasingly critical of facial appearance.[1–3] The explosion of digital photography, online avatars, carefully curated lighting, postproduction editing, photographic filters, and makeup has seen women seek facial plastic surgery to correct perceived flaws and set high expectations. This used to be taboo, but with a shift in societal acceptance, when women undergo excellent facelift surgery, it is increasingly considered empowering and may actually receive praise from friends and family. Amid the advent of more natural facelift techniques,

society has become more accepting of women who have had this surgery. Unfortunately, it still remains less accepted in men. Any hint of a facial rejuvenation procedure in a man might be met with dismissive judgment, disapproval, and intrusive questioning.[4] Many of the stigmata of more antiquated techniques may be covered in women with hair and makeup; however, in men, this is not a choice. This intersexual acceptance gap predicates the nuances of male concern at presentation to the facial plastic surgeon. While women seek restoration of estrogenic youth, such as arched eyebrows, a full midface, defined cheek profile, tighter jawline and flawless skin to ease makeup

[a] Dominic Bray Facial Plastic Surgery, 70 Harley Street, London W1G 7HF, UK; [b] Beverly Hills Center for Plastic Surgery, 465 North Roxbury Drive Suite 750, Beverly Hills, CA 90210, USA
* Corresponding author.
E-mail address: dominic@dominicbray.com

Facial Plast Surg Clin N Am 32 (2024) 339–351
https://doi.org/10.1016/j.fsc.2024.02.003
1064-7406/24/© 2024 Elsevier Inc. All rights reserved.

application, most men seek better neck and jawline definition associated with masculinity and strength giving less importance to other facial zones.[5,6] The demand for male facelift surgery is increasing.[7] Of utmost importance is a natural, unoperated appearance without the tell-tale signs of surgery (**Fig. 1**).[8] The dissatisfaction rate among male patients is higher than female patients for these reasons,[9] so surgeons performing male facelift and neck lift surgery should be cognizant of the causes of facelift stigmata and feminization in the male patient (**Fig. 2**). The surgeon must also be aware of the differences in soft tissue character and density that may lead to earlier failures and scarring when less thorough techniques are used.

Male Facelift Goals

1. Natural unoperated appearance
2. Acute cervicomental angle
3. Gonial angle definition
4. Softening of the nasolabial fold
5. Improvement in lower eyebag protrusion and lid–cheek transition
6. Midface improvements without overvolumization
7. Undetectable scarring
8. Unaltered or improved ears
9. Preservation of vascular plexus and facial hair

ANALYSIS OF THE MALE FACELIFT PATIENT

The remit of this article is facelifts for men, so we have omitted analysis of ancillary rejuvenation procedures such as brow lift and blepharoplasty. Depending on the patients' wishes and subsequent consent, planned modifications to the extended deep-plane procedure can be performed to curate a bespoke male facial rejuvenation. Described are some of the surgical stepwise techniques we employ to address the following

common male concerns with a focus on vectorial repositioning and deep contour definition (**Box 1** and **Fig. 3**).

SURGICAL TECHNIQUE
Anesthesia

The procedure is performed under local or total intravenous anesthesia in all cases. Local anesthetic solution of 50 mL of 2% lidocaine, 50 mL of 0.25% bupivacaine, 250 mL of normal saline, 2.5 mL of 1:1000 epinephrine, and 5 mL of sodium bicarbonate. Three milliliters of cyanocobalamin is placed as a colorant and indicator for safety. Tranexamic acid in solution is avoided in large flap surgery for risk of cytotoxicity and vascular compromise but may be given intravenously without much concern.[10]

MANAGING THE NECK

There have been several decades of debate about management of the aging neck.[11–17] Submentoplasty and platysmaplasty are performed in 90% of our patients and nearly all revision or secondary lifts, patients with severe laxity and banding, exaggerated midline descent that would not be corrected with facelift alone, lengthening of the cervicomental distance, laryngeal setback, low hyoid position, and submental deep volume contouring. Liposuction is rarely performed to avoid contour irregularities, darkening the skin and worsening of platysmal banding seen with overaggressive fat removal. Submental work is performed prior to lateral face and neck lifting prior in the majority of cases.

Subplatysmal Contouring

A short submental incision is placed along the internal mandibular border rather than the submental crease to avoid visible migration superolaterally

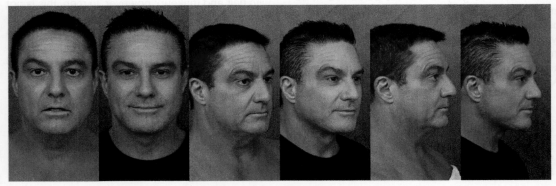

Fig. 1. Before and after deep-plane facelift and neck lift, brow lift, upper and lower blepharoplasties, and rhinoplasty. Restoration of masculine proportions and contours without tell-tale signs of surgery.

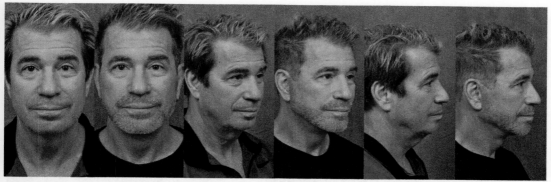

Fig. 2. Before and after deep-plane facelift and neck lift and chin implant. Neck and jawline definition are the predominant masculine goals.

with lifting. Following sharp incision, the supraplatysmal plane is opened with initial sharp dissection then blunt dissection. Dissection is carried inferiorly, stopping at the top of the thyroid cartilage and then continuing laterally to the extent of the retractor. Excessive caudal skin delamination is avoided to maintain a healthy blood supply to the watershed zone of the skin around the cervicomental angle at most 2 cm caudal to the hyoid. The medial or paramedian platysmal bands inferior to the hyoid have medialized over time and need to be moved laterally and vertically to restore proper function and position. The medial platysmal borders of the submental platysma are analyzed and pulled toward the midline to measure laxity. The borders of the submental platysma are then elevated using monopolar electrocautery followed by blunt dissection on the immediate undersurface of platysma keeping deep neck contents down.

Laterally, the dissection continues toward the lateral hyoid at the level of the lateral fascial sling of the digastric muscles. At this point, the submental and submandibular triangular fullness is evaluated, looking at the anterior digastric muscles, submandibular glands, and fatty lymphoid tissue in levels 1a and 1b. The central structures are more easily reduced and are thereby more likely to be over-reduced. When lying supine, the lateral compartment in the submandibular triangle may appear much less ptotic than when sitting the patient upright. For this reason, we recommend beginning reduction with the lateral tissues and remaining more judicious with the medial or central tissues. The central submental compartment should always remain slightly fuller than the anterior digastric and lateral triangles to avoid midline defects such as cobra or pseudo-cobra neck deformity. In most cases, we preserve the midline subplatysmal fat in its entirety.

Although the submandibular glands more often become ptotic than hypertrophic with age, there remains debate about whether or not to perform a submandibular gland reduction.[11,13]

Retrospective review of our cases reveals that imperfect outcomes or failures due to persistent gland or digastric prominence only occurred in 10% of patients prior to application of reduction techniques. For simplicity, in our practices, a submandibular gland reduction is performed if

1. The gland is pushing medially or inferiorly past the sling of the digastric.
2. The circumference of the neck at the hyoid appears too broad.
3. The gland has migrated into an anterior inferior capsule that would not reduce with lifting.
4. Volumetric reduction is required when the platysma would appear too weak to suspend the ptotic submandibular contents.

Box 1
Assessment of the male aging face

Lower eyelid fat pad protrusion and/or ectropion

Malar fat pad descent and the nasolabial fold

Buccal fat prominence

Jowls

Prejowl sulcus

Gonial angle and parotid size

Cervicomental angle and hyoid position

Larynx position

Thyroid cartilage projection and definition

Platysmal banding and neck soft tissue redundancy

Glandular, digastric hypertrophy

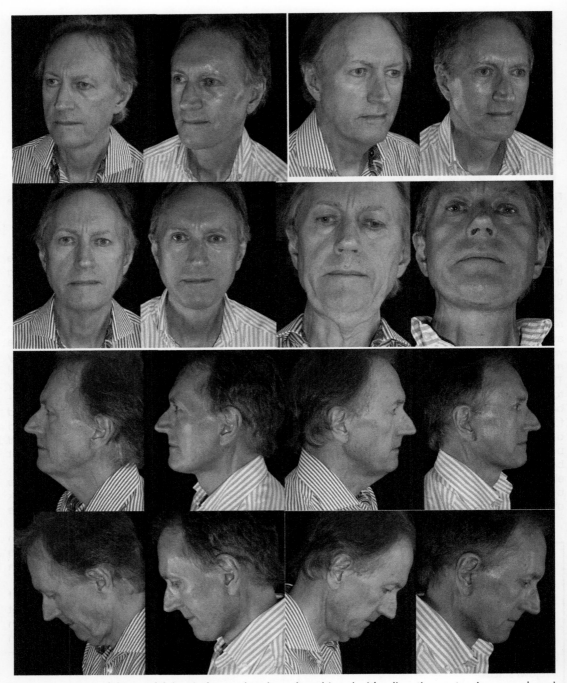

Fig. 3. Restitution of the youthful male face and neck can be achieved with adjunctive contouring procedures in the deep plane. A 71 year old gentleman exhibited all signs of male face and neck aging in **Box 1**. Following deep-plane facelift, deep neck contouring of ptotic structure, orbicularis oculi revectoring, and upper blepharoplasty, youthful unoperated masculinity is restored.

The latter can be assessed preoperatively but having the patient apply lingual pressure to their hard palate while seated and palpating the gland with and without platysmal contraction. The

creation of dead space in the submandibular triangle and submentum may provide less resistance to central plication and improve lateral lifting in many cases. The surgeon must remain judicious in volumetric reduction to avoid the appearance of excavation. We prefer reliance on lifting to obtain the majority of results.

To perform gland reduction, the medial and inferior portions of the gland are delivered from the capsule and injected with local anesthesia. The gland is then gently pulled medially to release it from the capsule circumferentially until only the stalk from the mylohyoid and floor of mouth remains. This area is then transversely transected using needle-tip electrocautery for cutting and bipolar electrocautery for ligation of ducts and vessels (**Fig. 4**).

Reduction is performed until the inferior gland is at level with the mylohyoid, cephalic to the hyoid, or deep to the mandible. The risk of bleeding increases with more posterosuperior dissection as the vessel caliber increases.[18] Our experience concurs with previous reports that 30% of glands have a perforator inferiorly.[19,20] In the combined 460 cases reviewed in the authors' practices, there have been no sialomas or subplatysmal hematomas without the use of neurotoxin, a subplatysmal drain or capsular imbrication. Although fluid collection may not occur, submental edema and submandibular gland induration might occur. These respond well to postoperative, scheduled manual lymphatic drainage and prior education that the dead space might take up to 12 weeks to contract and often improve for longer.

Fullness of the anterior digastric muscles might also be present. Plication of the digastric muscles is avoided in almost all cases to avoid medialization of the submental contents, although this is a valid option to infill previous midline reduction when needed or temporarily medialize glands to improve access. Complete digastric resection should be avoided to prevent any change in function or loss of support of the underlying mylohyoid

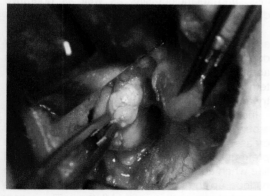

Fig. 4. Intraoperative view of the submandibular gland and the anterior digastric muscle through a 2 cm submental crease incision.

muscles. Anterior digastric reduction is performed by strip excision of the outer half of the muscle using bipolar electrocautery and/or scissors (**Fig. 5**).

The midline submentum should remain slightly fuller than the paramedian submentum as the midline will retract internally following platysmal plication and even more so when in the vertical position. Anterior digastric reduction may similarly increase postoperative edema in the submentum.

Cervicomental Angle

After the lateral volume has been addressed, the midline can be contoured. Midline banding and residual blunting of the cervicomental angle may be a consequence of platysmal laxity, hypertonicity, or an obtuse line along the deep cervical fascia. To address the cervical angle, the submental deep cervical fascia is grasped and pulled toward the chin, and a horizontal fasciotomy is performed across the prehyoid deep cervical fascia to expose the hyoid periosteum. This separates the infrahyoid and submental deep cervical fascia, permitting tighter approximation of the platysma during plication and sharpening of the cervicomental angle. Thyroid cartilage prominence can be sculpted if necessary, although this is desirable in men. Caution, however, must be taken to avoid overexcavating the prehyoid tissues in a male with a prominent larynx and thyroid cartilage unless a prominent Adam's apple is desired. The thyroid cartilage should be in the same anterior plane as the hyoid from a sagittal view. To avoid a prehyoid indentation in some patients, a submental drawbridge flap may be performed. The submental fat is transposed into the infrahyoid space by releasing the fat pad from the direction of the submental crease with a pedicle just above the hyoid. Following transposition, this fat pad may be secured with a suture or upon plication of the platysma in front of the fat pad.

Platysmaplasty is then performed using a classic platysmal plication technique.[21,22] Cadaveric studies have demonstrated that full plication platysmaplasty may limit the extent of vertical lifting in the face.[23,24] We believe that this effect is neutralized by limiting plication to submental platysmaplasty alone without infrahyoid extension.

To perform the plication, the platysmal edges are approximated in the midline using buried 2-0 polyglactin (Vicryl) sutures beginning in front of the hyoid advancing toward the incision with 3 or 4 figure of 8 mattress sutures or with a running vertical mattress.

Once the midline submental platysmal plication is completed, the cervicomental angle is palpated to check for midline banding. If a band is palpated,

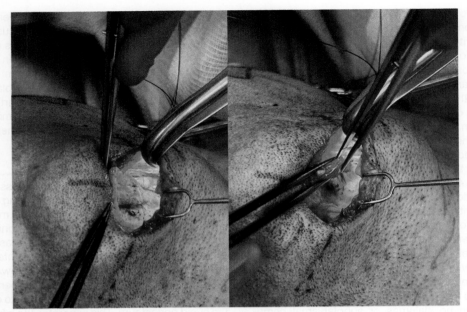

Fig. 5. Anterior digastric muscles are assessed for size and prominence and can be linearly reduced to sharpen the cervicomental angle.

a transverse or oblique myotomy is performed in the central 1 cm just inferior to the hyoid to release it. This is performed by retracting the platysma and incising the lower, medial third of the platysma using Metzenbaum scissors or monopolar electrocautery while keeping the deeper platysmal fascial layer intact to envelope the vessels and deep neck contents. The lateral two-thirds of the platysma should not be interrupted to avoid the loss of muscle integrity during the vertical lifting. If any dehiscence of the platysma has occurred, running plication may be performed to avoid herniation of deeper tissues.

Laryngeal Setback

The only benefit of infrahyoid platysmal plication is to posteriorly reposition the thyroid cartilage and larynx. This helps avoid prominence of the thyroid cartilage in patients where this is undesirable. Laryngeal setback can also have a profound effect on circumferential narrowing of the neck and by lengthening the cervicomental distance in those patients with a degree of retrognathia. The benefits of laryngeal setback or prelaryngeal platysmal plication must be weighed against associated limitation in lateral vertical facial lifting, which may be substantial. In most cases, we prefer to use the submental drawbridge flap, described earlier, to fill the infrahyoid indentation and soften the appearance of the thyroid shield from the lateral view.

EXTENDED DEEP-PLANE FACELIFT AND NECK LIFT
Marking and Skin Elevation

Incision markings are made followed by reference markings for the deep-plane entry point and Pitanguy's line. The entry design in our practices has been adapted using the "sailboat modification" to improve the positioning of the deep-plane entry point. This maximizes the composite area of the flap by reducing the delaminated skin at closure assuming the deep entry line will inset the temporal tuft incision angle. Limiting the amount of skin delamination may decrease ischemic effects on the distal flap including discoloration, beard hair loss, and telangiectasias as well as operative dissection time (**Fig. 6**).

It also improves volume along the zygomatic arch and lateral flap and lowers the chance of damaging the zygomaticus muscle complex. In addition, the superficial musculoaponeurotic system (SMAS) is thicker laterally providing easier entry and a better cuff for suspension.

Incisions are made with a No. 10 blade scalpel around the temporal tuft following the prehelical crease. The incision is placed in the immediate pretragal crease when present or in a retrotragal line when absent. The incision follows around the earlobe up the postauricular sulcus and crosses to the hairline as the mastoid flattens. The posterior limb incision follows the occipital hairline around 2.5 to 3.5 cm in most patients but can be

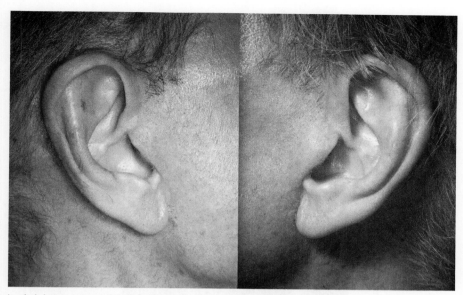

Fig. 6. Limited delamination of facial skin with the sailboat flap modification reduces skin stigmata of facelift trauma. Note no preauricular facial telangiectasia, but diffuse telangiectasia where a postauricular skin flap was raised. Scars are well concealed; earlobe shape and polarity are maintained; and hairline unaffected with careful incision planning and tensionless repositioning of facial soft tissues.

omitted in some. Incisions extending tangential into the occipital hairline are avoided to prevent hairline distortion and limitation in vertical lifting and redistribution.

Elevation of skin is performed with a No 10 blade scalpel in the subdermal plane leaving hypodermal fat on the reticular dermis to avoid violating the dermal vascular plexus or beard hair follicles, followed by scissor dissection and tension using the Anderson bear claw retractor and assistant counter tension. The postauricular skin is then elevated and connected to the facial skin dissection around the earlobe. The subcutaneous dissection continues using the Steven's Kaye scissors, bluntly spreading the supraplatysmal plane in the right hand while using a lighted facelift retractor in the left. The dissection is carried directly on the platysma to the midline. If a submental procedure was performed first, the 2 cavities may be connected at this point (**Fig. 7**).

Deep-Plane Transition

The sailboat line is marked on the SMAS deep-plane entry point and incised with a No 10 blade scalpel or monopolar needle with the dominant hand, while the other hand retracts the flap upward using a bear claw multiprong retractor. The deep plane is then entered and elevated beginning at the lateral border of the facial platysma where the risk is low.[25] Blunt dissection is performed with

vertical spreads of the Steven's Kaye scissors and continues anteriorly over the masseter, which is considered the deep glide plane or mobile portion of the SMAS–platysmal complex. Dissection ceases at the anterior border of the masseter and then continues inferiorly into the neck. Dissection is then performed on the underside of the platysma to elevate it off the tail of the parotid fascia inferior to the mandible. Dissection may continue inferior to the parotid tail where the platysma overlies the sternocleidomastoid muscle (SCM) and the external jugular vein. The decussation plane of fibers that exists between the lateral platysma over the fascia of the parotid tail is referred to as the cervical retaining ligaments. In the authors' experience, these dense fibers are found over the parotid and not over the SCM, as described in prior publications. A marking pen is then used to delineate the lateral border of the platysma and the cervical retaining ligament from the tail of the parotid, extending inferiorly to the external jugular vein, where the retaining ligament terminates as a mobile plane again (see **Fig. 6**). Blunt dissection using vertical spreads with the Steven's Kaye scissors is then used from the top down to release the cervical retaining ligaments off of the parotid tail, continuing inferiorly over the SCM and the external jugular vein where the mobile platysma elevates off easily. Great care is taken to avoid cervical facial nerve branch dissection and the small branches to the depressor labii inferioris under the platysma.

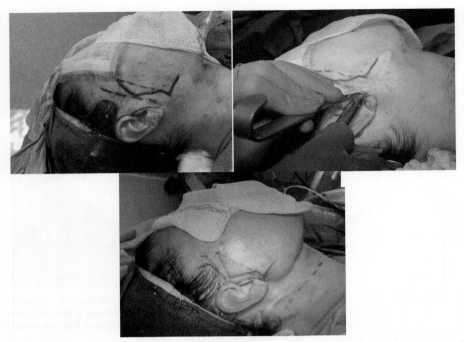

Fig. 7. Skin marking and sailboat modification of deep-plane transition point. Neck skin delamination is reserved for just 2 cm below the inframandibular border and the composite flap insets into the temporal tuft incision leaving minimal facial skin undermined at closure. We have termed this "Preservation facelift."

The midface dissection is performed next. The sailboat modification provides a thicker flap laterally that begins over the lateral extent of the zygomaticus muscles. Care must be taken to avoid transection of the lateral zygomaticus musculature, which may cause dimpling with smiling or smile block.[26] If partial or complete transection occurs, the muscles may be repaired with running absorbable sutures. The surgical plane in this region is contiguous with the plane of the platysma and contains the subdermal fatty fascial layer that we refer to as the fascial SMAS. Midface release is performed using blunt dissection to enter the sub-SMAS plane directly on top of the zygomaticus and orbicularis musculature. The orbicularis overlaps the zygomaticus muscle slightly at the point where the SMAS layer thins and tapers off over the orbicularis oculi. This zone is neither considered fixed SMAS (parotid region) nor mobile SMAS (platysma over SCM and masseter). Rather, a supramuscular dissection is performed to allow proper mobilization of the facial soft tissues without negatively impairing or affecting mimetic muscle function.

Orbicularis Retaining Ligament Release

The dissection can be extended in selective cases—which are identified and consented preoperatively to include lagopthalmos, lateral eyelid

bowing, postblepharoplasty ectropion, or aging scleral show—so as to incorporate a cuff of orbicularis in the SMAS composite flap by bluntly releasing the outer and inner lamellae of the orbicularis retaining ligament (ORL) in the suborbicularis space. Care should be taken to tangentially transect the orbicularis for 0.5 to 1 cm and only between 4 to 5 o'clock on the left side and 7 to 8 o'clock on the right side to avoid damage to surrounding facial nerve branches, namely, the temporal branch above and the buccal/zygomatic branches below.[27] Finger palpation of the suborbicularis space confirms full release to the arcus and gentle retraction on a Pitanguy flap clamp applied to the orbicularis–SMAS cuff confirms capture of the lower eyelid complex and cranial mobility of the lower lid margin to a more esthetically pleasing and youthful position, as well as deherniation of the suborbicularis oculi fat and softening of the palpebromalar sulcus (**Fig. 8**).

Midface Release

Dissection is carried in an inferomedially with blunt vertical spreads of the Steven's Kaye scissors or with a Trepsat dissector pointing toward the nasal alar base angled 10° deep. Tactile, percutaneous feedback helps maintain the proper plane of dissection as the SMAS release continues toward

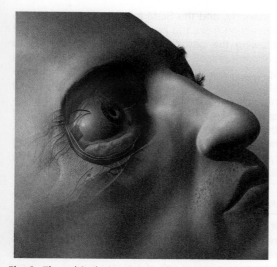

Fig. 8. The orbicularis retaining ligament (ORL) is a bilaminar structure. Safe tangential orbicularis transection and release of the ORL at defined points enable elevation of the midface en bloc and correction of postblepharoplasty or age-related scleral show and lateral lid bowing.

the nasolabial fold inferiorly and the nasal bridge medially. At this point, the buccal decussation zone is the only remaining area that needs to be released to connect the sub-SMAS pockets of the neck and midface. The lateral extent of the zone has been referred to as McGregor's patch or the zygomatic cutaneous ligaments.[28] This dense region of osteocutaneous fibers extends from bone to skin and anteriorly along the maxilla. Although release of this zone may occur at the level of skin or deeper along the bone, we believe the most effective release to occur at the level of the deep plane, allowing mobilization and repositioning of the fascial SMAS and superficial malar fat pad. Incision is performed under vertical counter tension sharply incising through roughly a 1 × 1 cm patch until palpable release of the reticular fibers is achieved. The transverse facial artery perforator exits in this region or anterior and inferior to the patch in 1 to 2 branches in most cases. When transected, bipolar cautery avoids the facial hematoma with the assistant watching the face for facial nerve stimulation. Elevation then continues anteriorly along the line of the parotid duct through the buccal decussation plane which contains the junctional interweaving fibers of fascial SMAS and platysma. These fibers must be released off the buccal capsule to permit full mobilization of the midfacial flap. Dissection typically terminates at the anterior extent of the buccal capsule, where platysmal fibers are seen diving deep and inserting

into the fascial SMAS. If the buccal fat is protruding or proptotic, it may be reduced. A small shelf is then made along the sailboat entry line, to provide a composite cuff for suspension. The facial flap is then repositioned and fixed via a cuff to the temporal parotid and tympanoparotid fascia (Lore's fascia).[29,30] Nonabsorbable or absorbable sutures can be used for the deep-plane suspension, as long as the sutures are positioned under no tension toward the individual patient's vector of greatest elevation. Confirmation of the greatest vector and position for suspension is achieved with palpatory feedback and the avoidance of bulging on either side of the incision rather than looking for the greatest effect of lifting remotely and distally. The proper appearance cannot be assessed with the patient swollen and supine. The vector of aging for that particular patient might not be the same on each side and is confirmed by passing a suture through the apex of the composite sail pulling the cranial end cranially, the lateral posteriorly with equal tension to lift the midface, jowl, and neck in vector of maximal correction. This demarcates the fixation point and if correctly designed should inset in to the 90° perihelical–temporal tuft skin incision, leaving minimal skin delaminated.

Gonial Angle

Once the facial flap has been suspended, the cervical retaining ligament patch is mobilized vertically, posteriorly, and deep in all X, Y, and Z dimensions to maximally manipulate and restore neck contours. Classically, the platysmal flap is posterosuperiorly lifted and sutured to the lateral mastoid fascia using a myotomy or transposition flap. Although this may provide a strong area for fixation, it may blunt the gonial angle in patients with a broad mastoid bone and fail to fully restore the submentum, as it most often will provide a less vertical vector than needed. To overcome the structural limitations of lifting over the mastoid, the second author (BT) has developed a technique—the "mastoid crevasse" which has substantially improved surgical outcomes in a large variety of patients (**Fig. 9**).[31]

The mastoid crevasse technique overcomes all natural limitations caused by variances in mastoid tip height and width as well as mandibular ramus height and position. The mastoid crevasse is opened by a vertical incision using needle-tip monopolar electrocautery along the anterior mastoid line. Incision is made down through the mastoid fascia to expose the anterior wall of the mastoid tip. The mastoid tip is bordered by the parotid tail anteriorly, the conchal bowl and ear canal

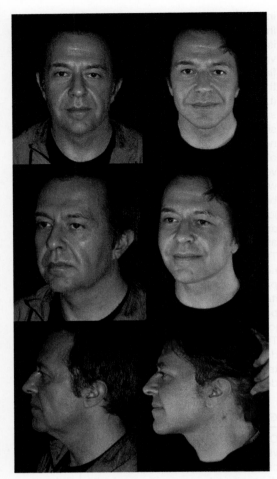

Fig. 9. Suborbicularis space dissection and orbicularis retaining ligament release incorporate lateral orbicularis into the SMAS–platysmal composite flap during deep-plane facelift. In some patients, this might obviate the need for lower blepharoplasty by using an orbicularis hammock to deherniate infraorbital fat pads.

superiorly, and the SCM inferiorly. Anteriorly, this dissection frees the parotid tail from the mastoid allowing the parotid and surrounding tissues to be compressed back into the deep pharyngeal space. Superiorly, the conchal bowl can be elevated very slightly to facilitate a more vertical repositioning of the platysmal cervical retaining ligaments, allowing a more substantial correction of the inferior neck and submandibular triangle. Inferiorly, the dissection stops at the SCM to avoid greater auricular nerve damage. The facial nerve exits the stylomastoid foramen 1 cm deep.

Parotid Reduction

If parotid hypertrophy is present, a minor tail of parotid reduction may be performed at this point to reduce the tail of the parotid, although this may introduce a minor risk of sialoma and should only be performed as needed. The fascia overlying the parotid tail is elevated reflecting the great auricular nerve within the fascia. A wedge of parotid can safely be excavated from underneath the retracted fascia. Parotid excision is limited to the anterior border of the great auricular nerve while avoiding any excision deep to the mastoid tip to avoid any heat dispersion to the facial nerve as it exits the stylomastoid foramen. Wedge removal provides increased collapsibility of the parotid and less resistance to platysmal lifting and inset of the parotid tail into the deep pharyngeal space. The fascia should be closed to lessen the risk of parotid gland exposure and potential sialoma. If sialoma occurs, treatment with a combination of bland diet, anticholinergic patches, botulinum toxin injections,[32] serial aspiration,[33] suction drainage, and/or compression with a bolstered gauze and silk net provides the compressive surface area to provide sialostasis far better than a net alone (**Fig. 10**).

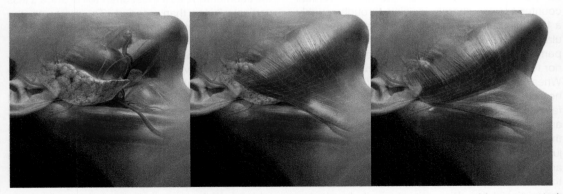

Fig. 10. The mastoid crevasse. Lateral platysma inset deep on to the anterior mastoid process enables true vertical platysma elevation, inframandibular border depth, and definition and contour creation of the mandibular ramus.

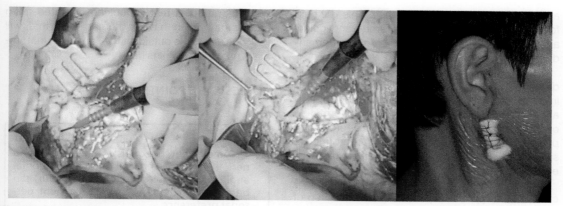

Fig. 11. (*A*) Dissection under superficial cervical fascia, reflecting the great auricular nerve forward enables hypertrophic parotid tail reduction to slim the lower facial third and define the ramus better. (*B*) Sialoma can be effectively compressed with a bolstered net, along with antisialogogues, a bland diet, botulinum toxin type A injection, and serial aspiration or drainage.

Lateral Necklift Crevasse Inset

Exposure of the anterior mastoid line allows inset of the platysma into the anterior mastoid rather than an onlay over the mastoid. This provides a better position of fixation with substantially improved gonial angle depth and vertical platysma movement. It is important to maintain continuity and integrity of the inframandibular platysma, which directly elevates the hyoid and submental contents. This also aids better encapsulation of the parotid gland and tail, slimming the lateral facial fifths, especially in patients with parotid hypertrophy.

The divided cervical retaining ligament condensation of the lateral platysma is sutured on the anterior mastoid wall. The placement should be as vertical as possible, extending deep to the conchal bowl. The inframandibular platysma is tethered deep to the gonial angle, which serves as a lateral pulley or fulcrum, which has a secondary movement against the lateral hyoid and tertiary pull against the chin. This results in a more substantial elevation of the hyoid as it now swings vertically to or above the level of the chin and mandibular border. With the hyoid in a more internal and superior position, a greater correction of the anterior digastric slope and bowing is achieved, with restoration of the submandibular triangle contents toward the floor of mouth, resulting in a negative vector submentum in many patients (**Fig. 11**).

Myotomy is limited or avoided unless tethering of the platysma exists across the span of the gonial angle. If needed, partial myotomy or fasciotomy is performed in the shape of the gonial angle,

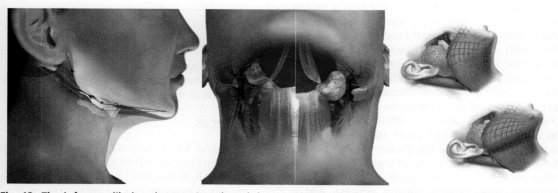

Fig. 12. The inframandibular platysma is tethered deep to the gonial angle, which serves as a lateral pulley or fulcrum and which has a secondary movement against the lateral hyoid and tertiary pull against the chin. This enables substantial vertical elevation of the hyoid to or above the level of the chin and the mandibular border. With the hyoid in a more internal and superior position, a greater correction of the anterior digastric slope and bowing is achieved, with restoration of the submandibular triangle contents toward the floor of mouth, resulting in a negative vector submentum in many patients.

avoiding a full myotomy or release. This will help form the shape of the vertical ramus and gonial angle while maintaining integrity of the inframandibular platysma (**Fig. 12**).

Contrary to antiquated beliefs, limiting skin dissection in the neck improves the gains achieved in skin quality. The true improvement in the appearance of the skin comes as a result of the formation of depth and contour rather than from stretching or pulling. There should be no tension on or around the soft tissues of the ear, assuring prevention of a pixie ear or telltale rotation of the ear.

Excess skin is then trimmed. A tension-free closure at all points helps ensure minimization of scarring.

Dermal sutures are avoided if possible to limit ischemia that may be caused by constriction of the dermal plexus as well as to avoid suture spitting that may result in atrophic or hypertrophic scarring. A No 7 French round drain may be placed in the neck bilaterally overnight. The suction tubing is mainly used to aid in redistribution of skin and to drain off blood-tinged, seromatous exudate rather than for actual prevention of a hematoma. Netting sutures are not routinely placed but saved for non-composite areas of the neck skin delamination in hypertensive patients at risk or excessive bleeders, and they are removed after 72 hours. A soft head-wrap is placed overnight with great care to avoid compression ischemia at the cervicomental angle.

SUMMARY

Men rightly fear the telltale signs of facelift surgery and have historically been less inclined to seek surgical rejuvenation of the aging face. The deformities of both tension and vector caused by superficial, nonligament releasing, tension-based SMAS techniques have made men a discerning facelift demographic seeking higher quality results today. As professional and social lives extend well into the sixth decade and beyond, men are an increasing subset of our patient base.[7] Using the techniques described in this article, we can deliver male patients predicable, unoperated outcomes, providing proper and impressive changes around the face, jawline, and neck. Structure is returned to such an extent that most patients perceive such a restoration as completely customized to their needs and restoration of their specific aging changes. While surgeons treating female patients primarily seek midface volume increase and a smooth ogee curve, when treating men we may be more focused on a strong, masculine jaw and neck line. Using more advanced techniques, as described in this article, all of these improvements may be universally achieved in both men and women without a fear of looking operated. Men and women both have a human face that will look natural on the outside if they are kept anatomically natural on the inside.

CLINICS CARE POINTS

- To some extent, the goals of male facelift and neck lift surgery (cervicomental angle, gonial angle, and submental and facial contour) can be anatomically customized to patient personal preference.

- Three-dimensional vectoring at the gonial angle is more important than maximal lateral distraction of the platysma in neck lift outcomes.

- Limitation of skin dissection may decrease ischemic effects on the distal flap including discoloration, beard loss, and telangiectasias, and operative dissection time and hasten visible recovery in male patients.

- Elevation of the cervical retaining ligaments allows for stronger mobilization of the fixed platysma of the parotid tail and provides a stronger density of tissue to suspend relative to weaker, more friable platysmal muscle.

- ORL release is a powerful addition to the SMAS–platysmal composite flap and can obviate the need for concomitant lower blepharoplasty in some patients.

- Any subplatysmal midline reduction necessitates equal lateral deep neck reduction. Failure to do so may result in a relative appearance of submandibular gland ptosis causing cobra or pseudo-cobra neck deformity.

DISCLOSURE

The authors have nothing to disclose. The techniques and methods outlined in this article are the opinions of the authors.

REFERENCES

1. Jacono AA, Talei B. Vertical neck lifting. Facial Plast Surg Clin North Am 2014;22(2):285–316.
2. Jacono AA, Malone MH, Talei B. Three-dimensional analysis of long-term midface volume change after vertical vector deep-plane rhytidectomy. Aesthetic Surg J 2015;35(5):491–503.
3. Jacono AA. Bryant LM Release and composite flap shifts to maximize midface, jawline and neck rejuvenation. Clin Plast Surg 2018;45:527–54.

4. Marten T, Elyassnia D. Male facelift. Clin Plast Surg 2022;49:221–56.

5. Stuzin JM. Discussion: a comparison of the full and short scar facelift incision techniques in multiple sets of identical twins. Plast Reconstr Surg 2016; 137:1715–7.

6. Bravo FG. Reduction neck lift: The importance of the deep structures of the neck to the successful neck lift. Clin Plast Surg 2018;45:485–506.

7. Aesthetic plastic surgery national databank statistics 2020. Aesthetic Surg J 2021;41:1–16.

8. Marten TJ, Elyassnia DR. Male facelift. In: Neligan, editor. Plastic surgery. 4th editio. Amsterdam: Elselvier; 2018.

9. Sarcu D, Adamson A. Psychology of the facelift patient. Facial Plast Surg 2017;33(3):252–9.

10. Yalamanchili S, Frankel AS, Talei B, et al. Wound healing complications with tranexamic acid: Not the silver bullet after all [published online ahead of print, 2023 Jun 2]. Aesthetic Surg J 2023;43(12): 1409–15.

11. Bravo FG. Neck contouring and rejuvenation in male patients through dual-plane reduction neck lift. Clin Plast Surg 2022;49(2):257–73.

12. Bravo FG. Reduction neck lift. Clin Plast Surg 2018; 45(4):485–506.

13. McCleary SP, Moghadam S, Le C, et al. Age-related changes in the submandibular gland: An imaging study of gland ptosis versus volume. Aesthetic Surg J 2022;42(11):1222–35.

14. O'Daniel TG. Optimizing outcomes in neck lift surgery. Aesthetic Surg J 2021;41(8):871–92.

15. Connell BF, Hosn W. Importance of the digastric muscle in cervical contouring: An update. Aesthetic Surg J 2000;20(1):12–6.

16. Connell BF, Shamoun JM. The significance of digastric muscle contouring for rejuvenation of the submental area of the face. Plast Reconstr Surg 1997; 99(6):1586–90.

17. Labbé D, Giot JP, Kaluzinski E. Submental area rejuvenation by digastric corset: Anatomical study and clinical application in 20 cases. Aesthetic Plast Surg 2013;37(2):222–31.

18. Cakmak O, Buyuklu F, Kolar M, et al. Deep neck contouring with a focus on submandibular gland vascularity: A cadaver Study. Aesthetic Surg J 2023;43(8):805–16.

19. Feldman JJ. Submandibular salivary gland bulges. In: Feldman JJ, editor. Neck lift. 1st edition. Germany: Thieme; 2006. p. 417–68.

20. O'Daniel TG. Understanding deep neck anatomy and its clinical relevance. Clin Plast Surg 2018; 45(4):447–54.

21. Feldman JJ. Corset platysmaplasty. Plast Reconstr Surg 1990;85(3):333–43.

22. LaFerriere KA, Paik YS. Complete corset platysmaplasty: Evolution of addressing the aging neck. Facial Plast Surg 2014;30(4):431–7.

23. Jacono AA, Malone MH. The effect of midline corset platysmaplasty on degree of face-lift flap elevation during concomitant deep-plane face-lift: A cadaveric study. JAMA Facial Plast Surg 2016;18(3): 183–7.

24. Kamer FM, Frankel AS. SMAS rhytidectomy versus deep plane rhytidectomy: An objective comparison. Plast Reconstr Surg 1998;102(3):878–81.

25. Jacono A, Bryant LM. Extended deep plane facelift: Incorporating facial retaining ligament release and composite flap shifts to maximize midface, jawline and neck rejuvenation. Clin Plast Surg 2018;45(4): 527–54.

26. Schmidt KL, Ambadar Z, Cohn JF, et al. Movement differences between deliberate and spontaneous facial expressions: Zygomaticus action in smiling. J Nonverbal Behav 2006;30(1):37–52.

27. Innocenti A, Dreassi E, Carla V, et al. Evaluation of residual neuromuscular intergrity in the orbicularis oculi muscle after lower eyelid transcutaneous blepharoplasty according to Reidy Adamson-s flap. Aesthetic Plast Surg 2020;(44):1577–83.

28. Duan J, Cong LY, Luo CE, et al. Clarifying the anatomy of the zygomatic cutaneous ligament: Its application in midface rejuvenation. Plast Reconstr Surg 2022;149(2):198e–208e.

29. Freeman BS. An Atlas of Head and Neck Surgery. JAMA 1974;228(12):1591–2.

30. Furnas DW. The retaining ligaments of the cheek. Plast Reconstr Surg 1989;83(1):11–6.

31. Talei B, Shauly I, Marxen T, et al. The mastoid crevasse and 3-dimensional considerations in deep plane necklifting. Aesthetic Surg J 2023;44(2):NP132–48.

32. Marchese-Ragona R, De Fillippis C, Staffieri A, et al. Parotid fistula: Treatment with botulinum toxin. Plast Recontr Surg 2001;107(3):886–7.

33. Auersvald A, Auersvald LA, Uebel C. Subplatysmal necklift: A retrospective analysis of 504 patients. Aesthetic Surg J 2017;37(1):1–11.

Direct Neck Lift for Men

Jeffrey T. Gu, MD, MS, Tom D. Wang, MD, Myriam Loyo, MD, MCR*

KEYWORDS

- Direct neck lift • Platysmaplasty • Cervicoplasty • Rhytidectomy

KEY POINTS

- Direct neck lift approaches, with limited dissection and fast recovery, may offer significant benefit for patients who may not desire full rhytidectomy.
- Disadvantages of the direct neck lift for the aging neck include the visibility of the incisions and scars as well as the limited area of the treatment in the neck.
- Direct neck lift surgical techniques address excessive skin and provide access to underlying submental and submandibular areas giving exposure to the underlying fat, platysma and digastric muscle, and hyoid bone.
- Patient selection, preoperative screening, and counseling are important to address in order to obtain optimal results during direct neck lift.
- The Grecian urn design with a Z-plasty at the level of the hyoid and platysmal plication is our preferred approach. An overview of many of the most commonly used direct cervicoplasty approaches is given.

INTRODUCTION

The neck is a critical component of facial aesthetics, as it plays a vital role in defining the jawline and overall facial balance. Submental fullness and laxity of the cervical skin are a common complaint of patients seeking aesthetic consultation. Many male patients present for evaluation of a "turkey gobbler" or "turkey waddle" deformity[1] and complain of redundant tissue in the submental area that rubs against the shirt collar or is pinched when wearing a necktie.

Patients often present with concerns that would benefit from rhytidectomy but may not desire to undergo a full rhytidectomy. Many of these patients may be reasonably well served by a direct neck lift. There are a multitude of limited direct excisional techniques to consider if submental fullness is the patient's primary concern. The advantages of a direct neck lift compared with rhytidectomy include shorter operative time and faster recovery. The disadvantages of the direct approach are inherent to the relatively limited area being addressed and visibility of the incision and resulting scar.

Direct excision of submental fullness and redundant skin offers an excellent alternative to rhytidectomy in many clinical situations, and many surgical approaches and techniques have been described. In this chapter, the authors provide an overview of direct submentoplasty techniques as well as clinical pearls to consider in the preoperative, intraoperative, and postoperative periods. All of the approaches described allow for excellent access to the structures deep to the skin and may incorporate additional treatment options as indicated to address the underlying musculature, fat, and skeleton. Given the degree of variation of submental fullness with which patients present, it is beneficial to be familiar with several different techniques to address the submental and submandibular areas.

Department of Otolaryngology–Head and Neck Surgery, Oregon Health & Science University, Portland, OR 97239, USA
* Corresponding author. Department of Otolaryngology–Head & Neck Surgery, Division of Facial Plastic and Reconstructive Surgery, Oregon Health and Science University, 3181 Southwest Sam Jackson Park Road, Portland, OR 97239.
E-mail address: loyo@ohsu.edu

Facial Plast Surg Clin N Am 32 (2024) 353–360
https://doi.org/10.1016/j.fsc.2024.02.004

DISCUSSION
Preoperative Considerations

Appropriate patient selection and preoperative planning are imperative for successful results. Skin elasticity, submental fat accumulation, and platysmal strength vary by individual and age and are responsible for the shape of the neck. The ideal cervicomental angle ranges between 90° and 105°, with the vertex at the hyoid bone and limbs extending tangentially through the gnathion superiorly and sternal notch inferiorly.[2] The effect of aging on the submental structures leads to changes of the skin, fat, and muscle. The skin relaxes due to degeneration of the collagen and elastic fibers and begins to hang beneath the mandible. With aging, some patients may develop an increase of fat deposition in the submental and submandibular areas, leading to a loss of the youthful neck contour. Furthermore, with aging, the platysma becomes flaccid, fibrous, and contracted, leading to varying amounts of platysmal banding.[3,4]

Many patients present for consultation desiring something less than a face lift to improve their neck. Patients must be counseled of the fact that all direct excisional techniques will involve a scar of the anterior cervical skin that may be visible, especially early in the healing process. The potential risk for hypertrophic scarring and need for additional procedures must also be discussed. In addition, the patients must understand the limitations to a direct neck lift approach, namely that the procedure is designed to address the neck and would not address facial rhytids.[5]

The most successful results are seen in healthy patients without systemic disease who have these soft tissue and structural characteristics—ptotic and loose skin and musculature of the neck extending no lower than the thyroid cartilage, minimal jowl formation, with favorable chin projection, a higher hyoid anatomic position—and are minimally obese.[5] The obese patient with heavy deposits of adipose fat along the jawline near the submental cervical area is a favorable candidate.

Physical examination should evaluate neck skin quality and elasticity, platysmal banding and laxity, amount and location of submental fat, position of the hyoid-thyroid cartilage complex, submandibular gland position, and mandibular/mental projection. Patients with more extensive laxity, adiposity, and platysmal banding may still be treated with direct neck lift with significant improvement but may require incisions to be extended to a lower, more visible portion of the neck.[6] Relative anatomic issues including submandibular gland ptosis may affect results and should also be considered preoperatively. Although it is possible to perform resections of the digastric musculature and submandibular glands, sufficient improvement may often be achieved with skin removal alone.[7] Additional considerations including placement of a chin implant may also be performed through the same incisions. Alternatively, a circum-occipital extended neck lift has been proposed, where incisions are placed posteriorly and excess skin is advanced posteriorly along the hairline. However, this technique is best for patients without significant submental liposis.[8] Furthermore, although there are several techniques to perform neck lifting without skin excision, such techniques require patients with minimal skin laxity and are beyond the scope of this article.[9–11]

General and systemic considerations are important to consider and manage appropriately. Ideal candidates have no systemic or complicating factors related to their healing ability or safety during elective surgical procedures and have established realistic expectations and goals. The direct neck lift approach is preferred by patients for whom the neck is the sole source of concern or by patients who are time constrained, risk adverse, or medically unfit for a larger procedure.[4] Anticoagulant medications including aspirin, nonsteroidal antiinflammatory drugs, and blood thinning supplements should be stopped. Tobacco or nicotine use should be discontinued and avoided at least 2 weeks before and after to surgery to reduce the risk of skin necrosis, but the patient should be aware that they are still at a higher risk of skin compromise. Tobacco consents describing that risk would be advisable for legal protection and to document informed consent. Further, it is important to counsel the patient that there would be a risk of hair loss along the incision length due to trauma to the adjacent hair follicles despite utmost care not to injure them. Direct neck lift may be performed on an outpatient basis and can often be performed with local anesthesia alone or in combination with intravenous sedation. We recommend placement of preoperative markings with the patient in the upright position before infiltration of local anesthesia. The displeasing aesthetics are more difficult to ascertain in the supine patient.

Direct Submentoplasty Techniques

In the following section, the authors review existing surgical techniques for limited direct submentoplasty. Different incisions will be reviewed. All of the approaches discussed allow excellent access to the structures deep to the skin and accordingly may incorporate various treatment options for the underlying platysma and digastric musculature, fat, and identification of the hyoid bone.

Elliptical Excision

The earliest descriptions of submentoplasty with elliptical excision were reported by Maliniak in 1932 and Johnson in 1955.[12] In their report, an ellipse of skin at or below the level of the hyoid is marked and excised in a transverse fashion. They advocate that direct elliptical excision can be combined with rhytidectomy as well as direct lipectomy and platysmal imbrication.[1] The primary disadvantage of direct elliptical excision is the possibility of contraction bands that may form from leaving excess skin in the lateral direction or a deficiency of skin in the vertical direction.[13]

Lazy-H–Shaped Incision

Morel-Fatio described the Lazy-H approach in 1964 with an incision design resembling an H lying on its side (**Fig. 1**).[12] Incisions are marked with two horizontal and one vertical incisions. The horizontal incisions are positioned with the superior incision in the submental crease or just inferior to it and the inferior incision sitting lower in the neck depending on the deformity. The vertical limb connects the superior and inferior horizontal incisions in the midline. Wide undermining is performed laterally to the vertical limb, and the lateral flaps are elevated and advanced toward the midline. Overlapping skin may be excised as the vertical portion is reapproximated and closed directly. Alternatively, a Z-plasty may be used to break up the vertical limb. Deeper structures of the submentum may also be addressed via this approach. Because the lateral flaps are pulled only in a horizontal vector, the Lazy-H–shaped incision removes excess skin in the horizontal direction and does not affect vertical skin length.

T-Z Plasty

Originally described by Cronin and Biggs in 1971, the T-Z plasty is a similar method of skin excision to the Lazy H–shaped incision except that the horizontal components are elliptical instead of linear (**Fig. 2**).[13] The incisions are designed with a superior ellipse at the level of the submental crease, followed by a vertical limb at the midline. Flaps are undermined lateral to the vertical limb, and excess skin is resected. The platysma is plicated down to the level of the hyoid. Submental fat between the anterior bellies of the digastric muscles may be addressed through this approach. Z-plasties are placed within the vertical portion of the lateral skin flaps with limbs no longer than 2 cm each. There is often a resulting dog-ear inferiorly at the level of the hyoid, which may be excised as a smaller horizontally oriented ellipse. The closure is recommended to be "quite snug," otherwise insufficient tissue has been excised.

W-Plasty

Ehlert and colleagues sought to further refine submental skin-excision techniques and proposed the submental W-plasty in 1990.[14] The incision is planned by marking the lateral extent of excess

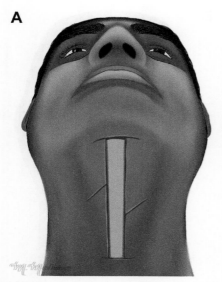 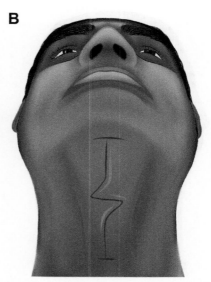

Fig. 1. Lazy-H–shaped incision. (*A*) An incision is made by marking one vertical and two horizontal incisions. The center segment of skin is excised and discarded. (*B*) The lateral flaps are undermined and advanced to the midline, and the incision is closed with a Z-plasty. The appearance of the incisions is that of an H lying on its side.

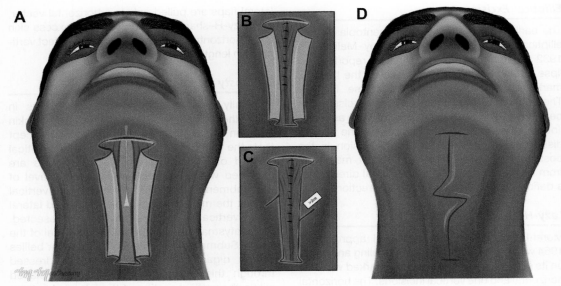

Fig. 2. T-Z plasty. (*A*) An incision is created by first excising an ellipse of skin in the submental crease. A vertical incision is then made inferior to the ellipse, and the flaps are undermined. (*B*) The excess lateral skin is excised and discarded. (*C*) Excess fat and platysma also are often treated at this step. (*D*) The vertical limb is closed with a Z-plasty. Dog ears at the inferior extent of the incision may be corrected with another elliptical excision.

skin. Horizontal incisions are marked at the level of the submental and the suprahyoid crease. At the lateral extent of excess skin, a vertically oriented W-plasty is designed with multiple arms measuring no longer than 1 cm each. The flaps are undermined laterally, and any excess submental fat is removed. A vertical strip of excess skin is excised as marked for W-plasty (**Fig. 3**). The

W-plasty is then closed in layers. Occasionally, dog ears may be present at the superior- and inferior-most aspects of the repair and may be excised by removing triangular portions of skin at the apex of the dog ear. The W-plasty disrupts the vertical portion of the scar and leads to a much less apparent midline scar, which is hidden within the shadow of the submentum.

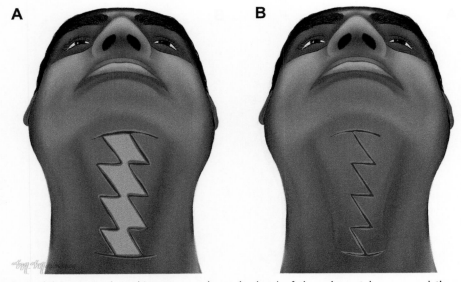

Fig. 3. W-plasty. (*A*) Horizontal markings are made at the level of the submental crease and the suprahyoid crease. The horizontal incisions are made, and a vertically oriented W-plasty is designed. The central strip of excess skin is removed, preserving the W-plasty configuration. (*B*) The W-plasty is closed.

Vertically Oriented Elliptical Excision with a T-Closure

Miller and Orringer described a vertically oriented excision of an ellipse of skin with T-closure in 1996.[15] An ellipse is marked at the level of the submental crease superiorly. Inferiorly, the incision may cross below the level of the hyoid depending on the severity of the deformity but usually lies above the notch of the thyroid cartilage. The elliptical incision is carried down to the level of the platysma, removing excess subcutaneous fat. Undermining is performed at the superior aspect of the ellipse and laterally for about 6 cm in a supraplatysmal plane. The platysma may be plicated at the anterior margins of the muscle to reduce tension across the skin at the incision site. Two acutely angled incisions are made at the superolateral aspect of the ellipse, and excess skin is removed. The resulting corners of the lateral skin flaps are advanced superomedially to close into the configuration of a T-shaped line (**Fig. 4**). The vertical limb of the T may be broken up with Z-plasties if needed, with the lateral arms of the Z-plasty measuring 3 to 3.5 cm in length and the transverse portion of the Z-plasty oriented within the suprahyoid crease. If the inferior portion of the vertically oriented ellipse is at or above the suprahyoid crease, a Z-plasty closure is unnecessary.

Bilateral Hemi-Ellipse

Hamilton described a limited submental lipectomy with skin excision in 1993 by excising two hemi-ellipses.[16] A midline incision is marked, followed by arcs diagonally oriented from each other in the configuration of a naval flag. The midline incision is made, and an arc of skin and subcutaneous fat is removed from one side of the superior portion of the ellipse, followed by an arc at the contralateral inferior portion of the ellipse (**Fig. 5**). The remaining flaps of the ellipse are widely undermined in a supraplatysmal plane. Platysmal plication and any appropriate fat removal are performed. The flaps are pulled laterally and closed with the resulting scar appearing similar to a Z-plasty closure.

Grecian Urn Technique

The Grecian urn technique was described by Farrior and colleagues in 1990 and has since been used with excellent results. As such, it is the authors' preferred approach. Markings are planned with a single vertical fusiform excision and horizontally oriented fusiform excisions superiorly and inferiorly. The vertically oriented ellipse of skin is marked by first pinching the skin together at the level of the cervicomental angle. The superior apex of this ellipse is positioned at the submental crease. The inferior apex is positioned at the level of the thyroid notch or extended further

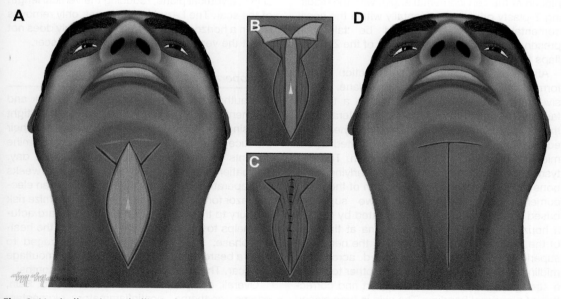

Fig. 4. Vertically oriented elliptical excisions with a T-closure. (*A*) A vertically oriented central ellipse of skin is marked and removed with the apex of the ellipse at the submental crease; the inferior point varies depending on the pathologic characteristics. (*B*) An acutely angled triangle of skin is then removed between the submental crease and the superior portion of the ellipse. Platysma and fat are then addressed. (*C*) The skin edges are reapproximated and closed. (*D*) The final closure is T shaped.

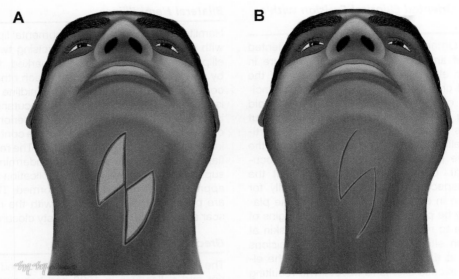

Fig. 5. Bilateral hemi-ellipse. (*A*) A vertically oriented ellipse is marked. A midline vertical incision is made connecting the apices of the ellipse. The superior portion of one-half of the ellipse is excised together with underlying excess fat. A similar procedure is performed on the inferior segment of the contralateral half of the ellipse. Once undermined, platysmal plication and excess fat removal can be performed. (*B*) Final closure leaves a scar similar to a Z-plasty.

inferiorly if needed depending on the amount of skin removal required. The superior and inferior horizontally oriented ellipses are marked at the level of the apices of the vertically oriented ellipse. A 60° Z-plasty with limbs measuring 1 to 1.5 cm is placed at the cervicomental angle, with the resulting Z-plasty oriented horizontally within the cervicomental angle. Care should be taken to preserve vascular supply to the tip of the Z-plasty flaps to avoid necrosis.

After incisions are created, dissection is performed laterally in a supraplatysmal plane. Excessive subcutaneous fat is removed in a tapered fashion. Dissection should be carried laterally until the free platysmal edges are identified. The medial edges of the platysma are then plicated in the midline from mentum to thyroid notch. The platysma can be suspended to the underlying hyoid bone fascia to increase the definition of the cervicomental angle. Alternatively, two superiorly based platysmal flaps may be created by making a horizontal incision in the platysma at the level of the hyoid bone on either side of the neck. The superiorly based flaps are rotated across the midline and imbricated over one another to create a strong sling for submental support and correction of platysmal banding. The skin is then closed in layers. The final incision seems similar in shape to an ancient Grecian urn (**Figs. 6** and **7**).

The Grecian urn technique has several advantages. The Z-plasty functions to reduce tension

across the skin closure and to visually disrupt the linear scar, allowing for further enhancement of the cervicomental angle. The width of the ellipse serves to reduce excess skin in a horizontal plane, and superior and inferior ellipses remove excess skin in a vertical plane, reducing the vertical length of the scar. The Lazy-H, in contrast, only removes skin in a horizontal plane and accordingly does not affect the vertical length of the resulting scar.

Postoperative Care and Complications

The authors recommend wrapping the neck and submentum with a secure and moderately tight dressing for 24 hours postoperatively. In their practice, they remove the dressing and examine patients in clinic on the first postoperative day. The patient is directed to avoid shaving for 2 weeks postoperatively and thereafter to use only an electric razor for an additional 2 weeks to minimize risk of injury to the incision. Fortunately, a beard actually helps to camouflage the scar during the healing phase; in fact, patients are encouraged to wear a beard for as long as possible to camouflage the scar. The scar fades over weeks to months.

Overall, complications are rare and mild. Pain, edema, erythema, postinflammatory pigmentary changes, infection, bleeding, and scarring are possible risks. The rate of hematoma in neck lift is approximately 3%, with risk factors including hypertension, male gender, and use of anticoagulant

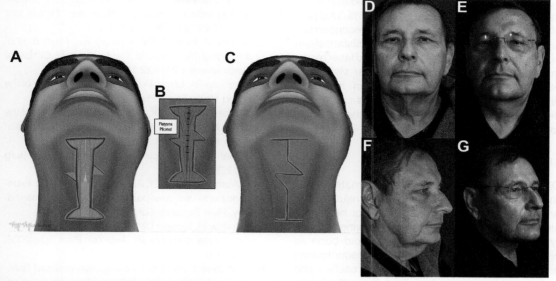

Fig. 6. Grecian urn technique. (*A*) A vertically oriented ellipse of skin is marked. The superior apex is positioned at the submental crease, and the inferior portion varies but may extend to the thyroid notch or below. Symmetric horizontally oriented ellipses are marked at the inferior and superior vertical ellipse apices. The final incision marking seems similar to an ancient Grecian urn. A 60° 1.0- to 1.5-cm Z-plasty is marked at the cervicomental angle. (*B*) Incisions are created, and undermining is performed in a supraplatysmal plane. The platysma is plicated to the thyroid notch. The skin is closed according to the indicated arrows. (*C*) The final closure results in scars generally well disguised in natural submental creases. (*D, F*) Preoperative frontal and profile views. (*E, G*) Postoperative frontal and profile views. Rhinophyma treated concurrently.

medications or supplements.[17] Drains and tissue sealants can be used in aging neck surgery. Hematomas after neck rejuvenation are rare and difficult to study. Nevertheless, current evidence has not demonstrated an advantage of using drains or tissue sealants to decrease the rate of hematomas. A meta-analysis demonstrated no statistically significant benefit from the use of tissue sealants in rhytidectomy.[18] A prospective, randomized controlled trial demonstrated no influence on postoperative hematoma occurrence by the use of drains in cervicofacial rhytidectomy.[19] If an expanding hematoma is encountered in the postoperative period, immediate evacuation of the hematoma and exploration of the operative site for hemostasis is essential to prevent airway compromise or flap

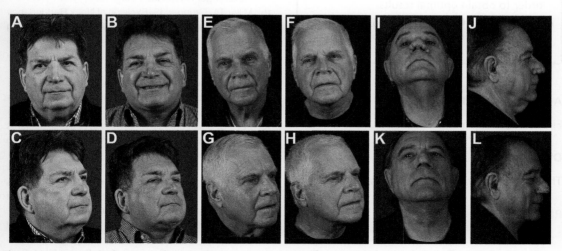

Fig. 7. Grecian urn before and after photos. (*A, C*) Patient 1 before. (*B, D*) Patient 1 after. (*E, G*) Patient 2 before. (*F, H*) Patient 2 after. (*I, K*) Patient 3 before. (*J, L*) Patient 3 after.

necrosis. Wound infection after rhytidectomy in general is rare with an incidence of 0.6%, and prophylactic antibiotics are not typically prescribed unless there is a concern for methicillin-resistant staph aureus colonization.[20] Scar revision and laser resurfacing can be used to minimize scar visibility if needed. Hyperdilute botulinum toxin injections directly into the scar every few weeks can further heal the scar, with minimal risk to the patient no matter the patient's skin type.

SUMMARY

Direct neck lift offers an excellent alternative to full rhytidectomy in men seeking neck rejuvenation and willing to tolerate a visible anterior neck incision. Surgical exposure to the underlying fat, platysma and digastric muscle, and hyoid bone as well as skin removal allow for neck recontouring and rejuvenation. Many surgical approaches and techniques have been described; the authors prefer the Grecian urn with Z-plasty at the cervicomental angle and platysmal plication. Given the degree of variation of submental fullness with which patients present, it is beneficial to be familiar with several different techniques to address the submental and submandibular areas.

CLINICS CARE POINTS

- Direct neck lift approaches may offer significant benefit for patients who may not desire full rhytidectomy.

- Patient selection, preoperative screening, and counseling are important to address in order to obtain optimal results.

- An overview of many of the most commonly used direct cervicoplasty approaches is discussed.

ACKNOWLEDGMENTS

Figures courtesy of Marielle Mahan, MD.

DISCLOSURE

The authors have nothing to disclose.

REFERENCES

1. Adamson JE, Horton CE, Crawford HH. The surgical correction of the 'Turkey Gobbler' deformity. Plast Reconstr Surg 1964;34:598–605.

2. Kamer FM, Lefkoff LA. Submental Surgery A Graduated Approach to the Aging Neck. Arch Otolaryngol Head Neck Surg 1991;117:40–6.

3. Shadfar S, Perkins SW. Anatomy and Physiology of the Aging Neck. Facial Plastic Surgery Clinics of North America 2014;22:161–70.

4. Adamson PA, Litner JA. Surgical Management of the Aging Neck. Facial Plast Surg 2005;21:11–20.

5. Thomas JR, Dixon TK. Preoperative Evaluation of the Aging Neck Patient. Facial Plastic Surgery Clinics of North America 2014;22:171–6.

6. Jordan JR. Direct cervicoplasty. Facial Plast Surg 2012;28:52–9.

7. Guyuron B, Sadek EY, Ahmadian R. A 26-year experience with vest-over-pants technique platysmarrhaphy. Plast Reconstr Surg 2010;126:1027–34.

8. Marshak H, Morrow DM. 'The stork lift': A circumoccipital extended neck-lift. Aesthetic Plast Surg 2008; 32:850–5.

9. Gryskiewicz JM. Submental suction-assisted lipectomy without platysmaplasty: pushing the (skin) envelope to avoid a face lift for unsuitable candidates. Plast Reconstr Surg 2003;112(5):1393–405.

10. Zins JE, Fardo D. The 'anterior-only' approach to neck rejuvenation: An alternative to face lift surgery. Plast Reconstr Surg 2005;115:1761–8.

11. Gonzalez R. The LOPP-lateral overlapping plication of the platysma. An effective neck lift without submental incision. Clin Plast Surg 2014;41:65–72.

12. Bitner JB, Friedman O, Farrior RT, et al. Direct Submentoplasty for Neck Rejuvenation. Arch Facial Plast Surg 2007;9:194–200.

13. Cronin TD, Biggs TM. The T-Z Plasty for the Male 'Turkey Gobbler' Neck. Plast Reconstr Surg 1971; 47:534–8.

14. Ehlert TK, Regan J, et al. Submental W-Plasty for Correction of 'Turkey Gobbler' Deformities. Arch Otolaryngol Head Neck Surg 1990;116:714–7.

15. Miller TA, Orringer JS. Excision of Neck Redundancy with Single Z-Plasty Closure. Plast Reconstr Surg 1996;97:219–21.

16. Hamilton JM. Submental lipectomy with skin excision. Plast Reconstr Surg 1993;92:443–7.

17. Batniji RK. Complications/Sequelae of Neck Rejuvenation. Facial Plastic Surgery Clinics of North America 2014;22:317–20.

18. Por YC, Shi L, Samuel M, et al. Use of tissue sealants in face-lifts: A metaanalysis. Aesthetic Plast Surg 2009;33:336–9.

19. Jones BM, Grover R, Hamilton S. The efficacy of surgical drainage in cervicofacial rhytidectomy: A prospective, randomized, controlled trial. Plast Reconstr Surg 2007;120:263–70.

20. Zoumalan RA, Rosenberg DB. Methicillin-Resistant Staphylococcus aureus-Positive Surgical Site Infections in Face-lift Surgery. Arch Facial Plast Surg 2008;10. Available at: https://jamanetwork.com/.

Facial Implants in Male Rejuvenation

Craig Cameron Brawley, MD, MS, MBA[a],*, Daniel D. Lee, MD[b], Philip Miller, MD[a]

KEYWORDS

- Male alloplast • Chin implant • Cheek implant • Jaw implant • Temporal implant

KEY POINTS

- Male facial alloplastic implants are utilized in augmenting and/or restoring bony and soft tissue volume.
- Facial alloplasts are most commonly used in the chin, but can also be used for the lateral mandible, midface, and upper face, especially when rejuvenation is the primary goal.
- Key factors when choosing the ideal implant and surgical approach include minimizing infection risk, size, customization, tissue resorption, stability, noncarcinogenic, and long-term aesthetics.

INTRODUCTION

Chronologic changes in facial structures play a predictive role in aesthetic surgery. Previously, these changes were thought to be primarily due to gravity and changes in the biomechanics of the skin, leading to rhytidosis; however, recent studies show that volume loss plays a key role. The resorption of bone, especially in the midface and mandible, has been proven in multiple computed tomographic imaging studies.[1–3] Male-specific, age-related facial soft-tissue volume loss has also been corroborated in a MRI study.[4] These documented losses of soft tissue and bone over time have changed the mindset of plastic surgeons to focus also on volume rejuvenation as a means to satisfy their patients.[5]

Volume augmentation can be performed through a variety of methods. Percutaneous fillers are the least invasive. The effects can be temporary and reversible, such as with hyaluronic acid, or have more lasting effects with products like poly-L-lactic acid, calcium hydroxyapatite, and others. A disadvantage of hyaluronic acid is that it is typically resorbed on the magnitude of months to years depending on the type, requiring further injections to maintain the effect. However, this can also be advantageous, as it gives patients a temporary experience of volume augmentation, and it can be dissolved if not favored. Another disadvantage is the unpredictable nature of a filler to augment a prescribed degree of desired projection. A disadvantage of longer lasting, non-hyaluronic acid products is their unknown risk with soft-tissue nodularity and the inability to easily remove the product.

Autologous fat grafting provides another augmentation method. This method is particularly popular for midfacial augmentation. Autologous fat grafitng can have a more lasting effect than fillers without the concern of foreign material. Disadvantages include unpredictable resorption of the fat after grafting, which can also lead to asymmetries, irregularities, and undercorrection.[6] In addition, weight fluctuation can pose a problem with weight gain showing fat hypertrophy and weight loss showing diminution of the result. Long-term survival rates are quite variable with reported rates between 20% and 80%.[7] There is also morbidity at the donor site; however, these risks are low.[8]

With both filler and autologous fat grafting, there are risks of vascular infiltration and occlusion from material injection, which can lead to devastating

[a] Department of Otolaryngology-Head and Neck Surgery, Division of Facial Plastic and Reconstructive Surgery, NYU Grossman School of Medicine, New York City, NY, USA; [b] Williams Center Plastic Surgery Specialists, Latham, NY, USA
* Corresponding author. NYU Langone Health, 222 East 41st St, 8th Floor, New York, NY 10017.
E-mail address: craig.brawley@nyulangone.org

Facial Plast Surg Clin N Am 32 (2024) 361–367
https://doi.org/10.1016/j.fsc.2024.02.008

skin necrosis. With hyaluronic acid fillers, hyaluronidase can be used to dissolve the filler and diminish this risk if acted upon early enough. Autologous fat and other fillers are not readily dissolvable, and treatment of occlusion and skin necrosis include additional, less direct methods of vasodilation to maintain perfusion. When working around the glabella and midface, vascular infiltration with these filler products also has the low yet catastrophic risk of retrograde embolization of the ophthalmic artery, leading to vision loss. This has most notably been described in Lazzeri and colleagues' review of 32 blindness events, with other studies reporting similar accounts.[9]

Alloplastic implants can yield a safe and predictable result to male patients seeking volume rejuvenation and augmentation of the face. These implants are made from a variety of materials, with advantages and disadvantages of each described in **Table 1**. Another issue that is posed with soft-tissue augmentation is their appearance as soft tissue rather than hard tissue after the procedure. In other words, if a bony chin augmentation is desired, fat grafting may just look like a fuller and rounder chin rather than a well-defined bony projection. The opposite may be a problem in the cheek area. Sometimes an undervolumized cheek could look even more skeletonized with an isolated alloplastic implant, but this is not always the case if the implant can span a wide enough area to compensate for enough volume loss where bony edges are not accentuated.

PREOPERATIVE PLANNING AND SURGICAL TECHNIQUES
Chin

Chin implants are typically inserted through either an intraoral transmucosal approach or external transcutaneous approach. The intraoral approach places an incision 2 to 3 mm anterior to the gingivolabial sulcus, which results in no visible external incision; however, there is a greater concern for postoperative infection. A recent systematic review including 3344 patients showed an infection rate of 1.1% intraorally compared to 0.5% from the external approach.[10] Unlike midface implants, saliva pools in a dependent gravitational position for this intraoral incision. Surgeons generally take the external approach when combined with other procedures like rhytidectomy.

Planning for the size of the implant can come from preoperative photographs, sizing, or simply experience. With the patient in the Frankfort plane, the ideal male pogonion lies at the 0 meridian line perpendicular to the nasion. Some surgeons have a sizing conversion ratio of their computed or printed images to actual augmentation. Others have a general sense of conversion or use sizers intraoperatively. Preoperative marking of the pogonion is made between the central incisors.

For the external transcutaneous approach, a marking between 1 and 3 cm at the submentum based on the type of chin implant used and surgeon experience. An incision is made down to the level of the periosteum. If a standard, smaller implant is used, then a central incision through the periosteum is typically performed to secure the entire implant subperiosteally. If an extended or anatomic implant is used, then a central portion of periosteum is left intact to prevent bony resorption, and the lateral limbs are tucked subperiosteally. The mental foramen and nerve are located inferior to the second pre-molar or 2.5 cm lateral to the midline, halfway between the distance of the alveolar ridge and inferior border of the mandible. Subperiosteal dissection should always be inferior to these structures to avoid injury. Anchoring sutures are generally used to prevent migration, which has already been mitigated by the subperiosteal placement.

Lateral Mandibular

Lateral mandibular or angle of mandible implants are usually inserted through an intraoral approach. A recent publication reviewing the literature found 4 studies with 57 patients total using this intraoral technique, with none of them having postoperative infection, and the only complication reported was unacceptable cosmetic outcome due to prominence of the implant.[11] There are fewer studies of lateral mandibular implants in the literature, and thus there are less data related to infection rates as compared to chin implants. In addition to these lower intraoral infection rates, the morbidity of possible marginal mandibular nerve injury along with higher scar visibility compared to the submentum makes the external approach less desirable.

A 3 cm incision is made lateral and parallel to the mandibular gingivobuccal sulcus, with the posterior extent of the incision starting at the second or the third molar.[12] An adequate cuff is left for watertight closure. The dissection is carried through the masseter and periosteum, and a periosteal elevator is used to develop a pocket around the posterior and inferior portion of the mandibular angle at the pterygomasseteric sling. The implant and pocket are then cleaned with antimicrobial solution once more before insertion. Depending on intraoperative assessment and surgeon preference, the implant can be secured to the periosteum with anchoring sutures or left alone. Others

Table 1
Facial implant characteristics in male rejuvenation

Materials	Other Names	Sites for Use	Biologic Sequelae	Advantages	Disadvantages
Organosilicone polymers	Silastic	Malar region Mandible Temple	Fibrous capsule	Chemically inert, hydrophobic, easy to sculpt, retains original shape	Bone resorption when subperiosteal, capsule contraction and possible dermal extrusion if too superficial
High-density polyethylene	Medpor	Malar region Mandible orbit	Extensive fibrovascular ingrowth	Biologically inert, non-biodegradable, no migration with soft-tissue ingrowth	Difficult to sculpt. Hard to remove due to significant tissue ingrowth
Expanded polytetrafluoroethylene	Gore-Tex	Malar region Mandible Temple	Minimal tissue ingrowth	Minimal inflammatory reaction, no capsule formation, easy to remove	Palpable, lack of capsule formation increases risk of migration, can lose their projection through compression over time
Methyl methacrylate		Temple forehead	Fibrovascular ingrowth	Morphologic plasticity for easy prefabrication	Allergic or autoimmune reaction
Mesh polymers	Mersilene Marlex Dacron	Mandible	Fibrovascular ingrowth	Can be folded or sutured for shape versatility	Can be difficult to remove, potential for implant degradation from foreign body reaction
Polyetheretherketone		Malar region Mandible Forehead	Minimal tissue ingrowth	Morphologic rigidity for bony augmentation, computer-aided design for precision	Rigidity can make it difficult to place with limited exposure

have utilized screws for stabilization.[13] The wound is then closed in layers using interrupted 3-0 chromic suture.

Malar Region

Midfacial implants, including malar, submalar, and combined implants, are approached from an intraoral, subciliary, or transconjunctival approach. The intraoral approach is typically most preferred due to the possible complications of ectropion or entropion from the lower eyelid approaches. The incision is hidden in the oral cavity and allows for wide exposure. Since it is not in a dependent position, salivary pooling is not an issue with this approach. Despite this seeming advantage, infection rates of 2.67% were reported in a recent meta-analysis consisting of 123 malar implant patients, which was a higher infection rate than all other facial implants reviewed.[14] This percentage is similar to a 1997 systematic review of 617 patients with malar implants, showing an infection rate of 2.4%.[15] The surgical approach for these studies was not stratified. It is especially important to practice aseptic techniques when inserting these implants.

Preoperative assessment of the type of malar region implant to use was best described by Binder and colleagues.[16] Type 1 deformity describes bony malar deficiency with adequate submalar and subcutaneous soft tissue. Type 1 deformity is best corrected with a malar implant for lateral projection. Type 2 deformity describes a soft-tissue submalar deficiency with adequate malar bone projection, best corrected with an inferiorly positioned submalar implant, typically superficial to the anterior maxillary sinus wall. Lastly, a type 3 deformity denotes both bony and soft-tissue deficiency, both corrected with a combined shell implant.

A 3 to 4 cm incision is made lateral to the superior labial frenulum and superior to the gingivolabial sulcus to allow for a cuff of tissue for a watertight closure. Dissection is carried down to the periosteum, and a periosteal elevator is used to create a tunnel lateral to the infraorbital nerve. The implant is placed with aseptic technique. All of these implants are either drilled in place, sutured to the periosteum, or have temporary external suture bolsters to decrease rates of migration. The incision is closed in layers.

Fig. 1 shows preoperative and postoperative pictures of a patient who received chin, lateral mandibular, and malar implants.

Temple/Forehead

Temple implants are typically silicone and approached from an incision in the hairline. When

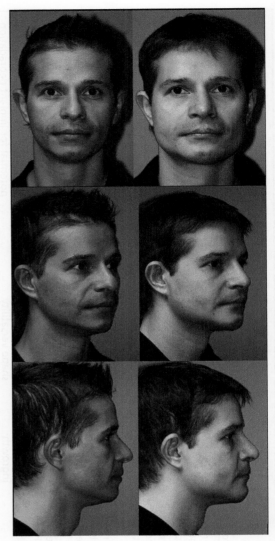

Fig. 1. A patient with decreased projection of the malar eminences, gonial angles, and chin. The preoperative photos on the left display a softened, ill-defined bony architecture, which is typically more feminine with traditional standards. Postoperative photos on the right display greater angulation of the jawline, chin, and malar eminence, ultimately creating a more masculine, square-shaped face. (*Courtesy of Phillip Miller.*)

combined with forehead implants, typically seen in east Asian cosmetic augmentation, methyl methacrylate can be used as the material and is often premolded before insertion.[17] This is performed with a coronal approach.[18]

An ideal, youthful temple can be described as a slightly convex curvature from the zygomatic complex into the forehead superomedially and hairline superolaterally. The region of temporal hollowing is different from the region superficial to the temporal fossa and includes the boundaries of the superior temporal line, temporal hairline, zygomatic arch, and lateral orbital rim.[19] Devolumization of this area, including atrophy of the dermis, temporalis, and temporal fat pad along with bony remodeling will lead to a gaunt appearance.[20]

For a simple temporal silicone implant without a combined forehead implant, a 3 cm incision is made in the hairline slightly anterior to the classic Gilles approach, and dissection is carried down through the temporo-parietal fascia to the level of the deep temporal fascia to mitigate injury to the temporal branch of the facial nerve.[21] A pocket is created anteriorly in the region of temporal hallowing, and the implant is inserted. The implant can then be anchored to the deep temporal fascia with 2 point fixation since it is fashioned in a gliding plane.

DISCUSSION

Alloplastic implants have many advantages. The material is predictable after insertion with much less risk of nodularity when compared to fillers and fat grafting. Alloplasts are long-term solutions that do not require repeat procedures like fillers; however, fillers can be used first to give the patient a preview before committing to a permanent alloplastic measure. There is a higher risk of infection in the immediate postoperative period with alloplastic implants, but this can be diminished with approach and sterile technique. These implants can be inserted with local anesthesia, sedation, or under general anesthesia if in conjunction with other procedures. They can be sized preoperatively with attention to patient photos or adjusted intraoperatively with different sizers. They can also be manipulated with fine trimming by the surgeon. The volume loss from the surrounding tissue over time is minimal, if any, making it an ideal permanent solution. The 3 most commonly used implant materials for facial augmentation are organosilicone polymers, expanded polytetrafluoroethylene, and high-density polyethylene.[22] For mandibular augmentation, organosilicone is generally considered ideal in that the material is firm yet flexible in placement, can be carved for fine tuning, stable due to encapsulation, has minimal-to-no loss of projection over time, and is easily removed.[23]

Infection, one of the highest concerns from the surgeon's perspective, varies between implant location and approach. Implant material further impacts infection risk. This was recently reviewed by Oliver and colleagues, with mersilene mesh having the highest infection rate of 3.38% from a total of 533 patients, followed by polytetrafluoroethylene at 2.86% in 35 patients, methyl methacrylate at 2.33% in 535 patients, and silicone at 1.58% in 443 patients.[14] In the same study, implant migration was highest with silicone (0.9%), wound dehiscence was highest with high-density polyethylene (0.78%), and hematoma was highest with methyl methacrylate (5.98%).

Though many infection risk mitigation strategies have been described, few have been proven in prospective trials. Implant soaking with antibiotic irrigation before insertion is a common practice, typically with gentamycin, bacitracin, or fluoroquinolone antibiotics. Alternatively, implant soaking in dilute povidone–iodine solution has been described. A new pair of surgical gloves can be donned before direct contact with the implant, and the antimicrobial irrigation can also be instilled into the surgical pocket. Intraoperative antibiotics are used similarly to most head-and-neck procedures. Some surgeons use a week-long course of oral antibiotics after implantation.

Other postoperative care includes a compression dressing for chin augmentation, typically with micropore tape. A head wrap can be used for upper and midface implants. These compression dressings for 24 hours are helpful to prevent hematoma and seroma formation. Chlorhexidine mouthwash is used for 1 week if an intraoral approach was performed. If signs of infection begin, a new course of oral antibiotics or addition of a new antibiotic should be trialed. If the infection continues despite medical intervention, explantation should be performed. The capsule produced around silicone implants makes medical management difficult with superimposed biofilm, and capsule is postulated to be why late onset infection is more prominent in silicone.[22] It is thought that high-density polyethylene could have an earlier rate of infection due to its porous nature, acting as a nidus for bacterial growth.[24]

Other risks of alloplastic implants include extrusion, migration, and general patient dissatisfaction. Extrusion is more likely with inadequate tissue/flap thickness and coverage, damaged tissue in the setting of radiation, and increased incision tension over the overlying tissue from large implant sizing.[25] A systematic review by Rubin and colleagues showed that the overall extrusion rate for malar and chin implants was less than 0.5%.[15] Migration can be reduced by intraoperative fixation first and foremost. Other techniques used to minimize migration risk are appropriate pocket dissection, choice of the proper implant size, subperiosteal insertion, and choice of appropriate anatomic shapes.[25] The highest rate of migration is seen in the mandible (1.08%), and the highest rate of poor cosmetic outcome is seen in the frontal (5.2%) and malar (4%) regions.[14]

Aging facial skeleton changes in men and women include mandibular height and length decrease, mandibular angle increases, and maxillary angle decreases.[3] Due to these similarities between genders, surgeons should anticipate these changes but always take a comprehensive history when a male patient presents for aging facial augmentation to completely elicit his concerns. Male patients typically have a greater concern about their lower and midface compared to women who are typically concerned with their upper face.[26] Without considering age, the lower face of men differ from women with a larger bigonial distance, more acute gonial angle, and a more squared and projected chin.[27] Mandibular and malar alloplastic augmentation will give them a more defined, youthful, and masculine lower and midface.

SUMMARY

Alloplastic implants used in male facial rejuvenation can provide a safe and lasting result. Trends in the male aging facial skeleton, baseline sexual dimorphism, thorough examination, and comprehensive discussion of desired results are key when devising a surgical plan with the patient. Familiarity of alloplastic materials, surgical approach, and anticipated complications are imperative for success.

CLINICS CARE POINTS

- Alloplastic implants are long-term solutions to bony and soft-tissue deformities in male facial rejuvenation
- Different materials can be used, with organosilicone polymers being the most utilized in the aesthetic practice
- There are different rates of infection based on the location of the alloplast, material, and surgical approach
- Traditional masculine appearances, changes with aging, and patient-specific desires should all be integrated in the preoperative planning

DISCLOSURE

Nothing to disclose.

REFERENCES

1. Paskhover B, Durand D, Kamen E, et al. Patterns of change in facial skeletal aging. JAMA Facial Plast Surg 2017;19(5):413–7.
2. Richard MJ, Morris C, Deen BF, et al. Analysis of the anatomic changes of the aging facial skeleton using computer-assisted tomography. Ophthalmic Plast Reconstr Surg 2009;25(5):382–6.
3. Shaw RB Jr, Katzel EB, Koltz PF, et al. Aging of the facial skeleton: aesthetic implications and rejuvenation strategies. Plast Reconstr Surg 2011;127(1):374–83.
4. Wysong A, Kim D, Joseph T, et al. Quantifying soft tissue loss in the aging male face using magnetic resonance imaging. Dermatol Surg 2014;40(7):786–93.
5. Lam SM. A new paradigm for the aging face. Facial Plast Surg Clin North Am 2010;18(1):1–6.
6. Cuzalina A, Guerrero AV. Complications in Fat Grafting. Atlas Oral Maxillofac Surg Clin North Am 2018;26(1):77–80.
7. Niechajev I, Sevcuk O. Long-term results of fat transplantation: clinical and histologic studies. Plast Reconstr Surg 1994;94(3):496–506.
8. Bellini E, Grieco MP, Raposio E. The science behind autologous fat grafting. Ann Med Surg (Lond) 2017;24:65–73.
9. Lazzeri D, Agostini T, Figus M, et al. Blindness following cosmetic injections of the face. Plast Reconstr Surg 2012;129(4):995–1012.
10. Oranges CM, Grufman V, di Summa PG, et al. Chin Augmentation Techniques: A Systematic Review. Plast Reconstr Surg 2023;151(5):758e–71e.
11. Rojas YA, Sinnott C, Colasante C, et al. Facial Implants: Controversies and Criticism. A Comprehensive Review of the Current Literature. Plast Reconstr Surg 2018;142(4):991–9.
12. Terino EO, Edwards MC. Customizing jawlines: the art of alloplastic premandible contouring. Facial Plast Surg Clin North Am 2008;16(1):99–122, vi.
13. Al-Jandan B, Marei HF. Mandibular angle augmentation using solid silicone implants. Dental and Medical Problems 2018;55(4):367–70.
14. Oliver JD, Eells AC, Saba ES, et al. Alloplastic Facial Implants: A Systematic Review and Meta-Analysis on Outcomes and Uses in Aesthetic and Reconstructive Plastic Surgery. Aesthetic Plast Surg 2019;43(3):625–36.
15. Rubin JP, Yaremchuk MJ. Complications and toxicities of implantable biomaterials used in facial reconstructive and aesthetic surgery: a comprehensive review of the literature. Plast Reconstr Surg 1997;100(5):1336–53.
16. Binder WJ, Azizzadeh B. Malar and submalar augmentation. Facial Plast Surg Clin North Am 2008;16(1):11–32.

17. Hirohi T, Nagai K, Ng D, et al. Integrated Forehead and Temporal Augmentation Using 3D Printing-Assisted Methyl Methacrylate Implants. Aesthet Surg J 2018;38(11):1157–68.

18. Chao JW, Lee JC, Chang MM, et al. Alloplastic Augmentation of the Asian Face: A Review of 215 Patients. Aesthet Surg J 2016;36(8):861–8.

19. Huang RL, Xie Y, Wang W, et al. Anatomical Study of Temporal Fat Compartments and its Clinical Application for Temporal Fat Grafting. Aesthet Surg J 2017;37(8):855–62.

20. Othman S, Cohn JE, Burdett J, et al. Temporal Augmentation: A Systematic Review. Facial Plast Surg 2020;36(3):217–25.

21. Rihani J. Aesthetics and Rejuvenation of the Temple. Facial Plast Surg 2018;34(2):159–63.

22. Patel K, Brandstetter K. Solid implants in facial plastic surgery: potential complications and how to prevent them. Facial Plast Surg 2016;32(05):520–31.

23. Papel ID, Frodel JL, Holt GR. Facial plastic and reconstructive surgery. New York: Thieme; 2016.

24. Berghaus A, Stelter K. Alloplastic materials in rhinoplasty. Curr Opin Otolaryngol Head Neck Surg 2006; 14(4):270–7.

25. Cuzalina LA, Hlavacek MR. Complications of facial implants. Oral Maxillofac Surg Clin North Am 2009; 21(1):91–104. vi-vii.

26. Brissett AE, Hilger PA. Male face-lift. Facial Plast Surg Clin 2005;13(3):451–8.

27. Straughan DM, Yaremchuk MJ. Improving male chin and mandible eesthetics. Clin Plast Surg 2022;49(2): 275–83.

Asian Male Blepharoplasty and Rhinoplasty

John W. Frederick, MD[a], Jae Kim, MD[b], Donald B. Yoo, MD[c],*

KEYWORDS

- Male blepharoplasty • Asian blepharoplasty • Male asian blepharoplasty
- Sub-brow blepharoplasty • Male rhinoplasty • Asian rhinoplasty • Male asian rhinoplasty
- Rib cartilage

KEY POINTS

- More Asian males seek cosmetic surgery than ever before.
- Asian male blepharoplasty should avoid dramatic change as much as possible, especially for older patients.
- Asian male rhinoplasty requires an understanding of the unique anatomy: a short nasal septum, short nasal bones, and thick nasal skin.
- Clear operative goals must be discussed, preferably with computer morphing. Dorsal augmentation rhinoplasty will likely be required.

INTRODUCTION

More male patients are seeking out cosmetic surgery than ever before, and it is especially true for the Asian male population, both in the West and in Asia. Trends across the Asian continent show increasing proportions of males seeking out esthetic treatment, from 12% in 2005 to 2009 to 19% in 2010 to 2014.[1] Contributing factors for Asian male patients include increased affluence, desire to invest in self or enhance self-confidence, and to some degree, external factors including peer pressure, advertising/celebrity influence, or recommendation from family and friends.

Over the past 25 or so years, the Korean wave, aka *Hallyu* (Korean: 한류), has given rise to the inexorable spread of K-pop and K-dramas, and with it, the ideal of an esthetic image, which is a key economic asset for South Korea. Along with this phenomenon of *Hallyu*, there are more Asian males in popular culture, many of whom have had esthetic procedures and plastic surgery. It is

not unusual for them to have "little tuckups" on a regular basis. They have hordes of fans across the world, both male and female, who admire their physical appearance as a part of the cultural brand and product. Now more than ever, there is decreased stigma and increased demand for plastic surgery among Asian males.

ASIAN MALE BLEPHAROPLASTY

A large online questionnaire across 5 major East Asian countries found that the most performed surgical procedure is Asian blepharoplasty (except in South Korea, where rhinoplasty is the top procedure), and for those who have no prior experience with plastic surgery, the top considered surgery is Asian blepharoplasty. While the data are not divided between male and female subsets, almost 40% of the total respondents were male, indicating an increased interest in plastic surgery.[2]

Like the female Asian upper eyelid, the male Asian upper eyelid often has a skin-levator relationship where the aponeurosis attachment to

a Department of Facial Plastic Surgery, Nassif Plastic Surgery, 120 South Spalding Drive Suite 301, Beverly Hills, CA 90212, USA; b Department of Facial Plastic Surgery, 10721 Main Street Suite 205, Fairfax, VA 22030, USA; c Department of Facial Plastic Surgery, HALO Beverly Hills Plastic Surgery & Med Spa, 433 North Camden Drive Suite 970, Beverly Hills, CA 90210, USA
* Corresponding author.
E-mail address: info@donyoomd.com

Facial Plast Surg Clin N Am 32 (2024) 369–381
https://doi.org/10.1016/j.fsc.2024.03.005

the upper eyelid skin is weak, thin, or altogether absent. As a result, the central or preaponeurotic fat extends inferiorly over the tarsal plate toward the ciliary margin, especially for younger patients whose upper eyelids appear fuller. Many Asian males have inconsistent eyelid creases, and some have a monolid.

During consultation, the patient's concerns and goals may not be so straightforward. Some patients come to the surgical consultation "because my wife/mother told me" or "because I look tired," but it may require some effort on the part of the surgeon to translate that into a definitive surgical plan that is consistent with the patient's esthetic goals. A major factor to consider in the evaluation and surgical management of the Asian male upper eyelid is age.

Surgical Approach for Younger Male Asian Blepharoplasty

The upper eyelids of younger Asian male patients, especially those without defined supratarsal creases, exhibit extra fullness. This shape can be indicative of excess suborbicularis fat, as well as preaponeurotic fat descending past the level of the distal levator aponeurosis toward the ciliary margin. The amount of desired eyelid show among younger Asian male patients is usually minimal. Therefore, a single incision without removal of upper eyelid skin to establish the supratarsal crease is sometimes sufficient to achieve the desired esthetic result. While there is utility in some cases for crease formation using the suture technique through partial incisions or multiple stab incisions, the author (JK) does not use that approach. That technique would not address the pretarsal upper eyelid fullness due to the suborbicularis fat or preaponeurotic fat, and it could lead to an undesirable sausagelike appearance for a prolonged period of time. If there is extra upper eyelid skin, a small amount, usually less than 5 mm wide, can be removed.

Using a full incision (**Fig. 1**), the surgeon is able to create a supratarsal crease and decrease pretarsal fullness due to orbicularis hypertrophy, suborbicularis fat, excess preaponeurotic fat, or a combination. The full incision also allows for correction of ptosis using the levator advancement technique. There are many described techniques of creating the supratarsal crease, most of which involve suturing skin and/or orbicularis to the distal levator aponeurosis and/or superior tarsal plate. The merits and limitations of these techniques have been described elsewhere.[3] If the patient has a double eyelid crease that is somewhat consistent, crease formation sutures may not be

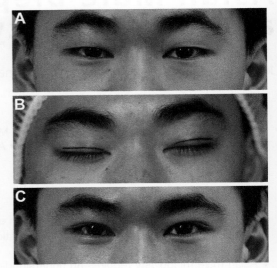

Fig. 1. This 19-year-old Chinese male presented for Asian upper blepharoplasty. He desired natural brighter eyes and improvement of entropion. Frontal view photos are shown at the preoperative visit (*A*), intraoperative markings (*B*), and 5-month postoperative view (*C*). This patient's upper eyelids lacked a supratarsal crease, and there was evidence of blepharoptosis along with entropion. He underwent full-incision upper blepharoplasty with supratarsal crease formation and ptosis repair with levator advancement. The full surgical incisions were made 5 mm above the ciliary margins. Of note, preaponeurotic fat was not removed. Five months after surgery, consistent low, natural eyelid creases are noted, along with a brighter appearance to the eyes.

required. Instead, they may unnecessarily weigh down the levator apparatus, leading to postoperative ptosis and prolonged swelling, which can be debilitating for the Asian male patient.

Like younger Asian females, younger Asian males may request lengthening or shaping of the horizontal palpebral fissures with lateral canthoplasty, medial epicanthoplasty, or both. Techniques for these procedures have been described elsewhere.[4,5]

Surgical Approach for the Older Male Asian Blepharoplasty

The upper eyelids of older Asian male patients tend to feature significant atrophy of upper eyelid fat, both suborbicularis and preaponeurotic. In some cases, there may be little to no preaponeurotic fat below the level of Whitnall's ligament, giving a hollower appearance, as well as the illusion of a high upper eyelid crease at or near the level of the supraorbital rim. In these cases, surgery via a supratarsal incision approach, with creation or reinforcement of a supratarsal crease, can lead to a quite different and unnatural appearance.

There are significant psychological ramifications of a sudden change in an older Asian male's appearance. When the older Asian male patient has known himself to look a certain way for his entire life, adjusting to a change in his appearance may be very challenging.[6] During presurgical consultation, a larger proportion of older Asian male patients may not say that they want a double eyelid, or they may say outright that they do not want it. Often the main concern is for their eyes to look less tired or droopy, regardless of whether they have a defined supratarsal crease.

The recommended surgical technique instead is excision of extra upper eyelid skin via a sub-brow approach. The patient's eyebrow position and thickness must be taken into account, and a sub-brow scar can be more noticeable than an extended supratarsal scar. However, with beveled incisions and meticulous tension-free skin closure, the sub-brow scar is less noticeable in the end than most patients expect. With older Asian males, lateral hooding of the upper eyelids is more prominent than central or medial hooding, and the sub-brow approach is ideal for patients with this concern. When removing excess lateral upper eyelid skin with a traditional supratarsal approach, the resulting scar must extend past the lateral canthus, which may be more conspicuous. The other concern with supratarsal skin excision is that when the dermatochalasis is severe and more than 7 mm of skin must be removed, the sub-brow skin above the incision can appear bulky, swollen, and unnatural (**Fig. 2**) because it is significantly thicker than the pretarsal eyelid skin in Asian male patients.[7] If the eyebrows are thin, treatments including micro-blading, eyebrow tattoo, or eyebrow transplantation may be worth considering several months after blepharoplasty to hide the sub-brow scars. Other surgical options include lateral browlift using temporal incisions or skin-only supratarsal upper blepharoplasty.

For the sub-brow upper blepharoplasty in the Asian male, the author determines the amount of skin removal as follows. The patient is seated upright in front of a mirror. Holding a ruler vertically in line with the lateral brow apex, the surgeon raises the patient's eyebrow to the point where the patient is satisfied with the amount of upper eyelid show. The distance is measured, and surgical markings are prepared with the amount of sub-brow skin to be removed (**Fig. 3**). Depending on the patient's natural eyebrow position, the total remaining skin between the ciliary margin and the brow after skin excision should be 24 to 28 mm to create the desired result.

Many older Asian male patients are accustomed to lifting their eyebrows to open their eyes; they

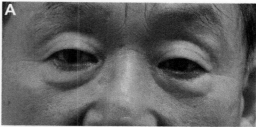
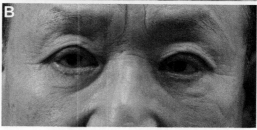

Fig. 2. This 63-year-old Korean male presented for Asian upper blepharoplasty and lower blepharoplasty. His preoperative photo (*A*) shows severe dermatochalasis extending laterally past the lateral canthus, as well as a lack of supratarsal crease and significant hollowing. Given his anatomic features, a sub-brow blepharoplasty would have been the preferred technique, but he underwent traditional supratarsal upper blepharoplasty. Three months later (*B*), the patient's appearance remains harsh and unnatural.

have been opening their eyes that way for so long. What may occur after sub-brow blepharoplasty is that their brow position may become lower, as a result of decreased use of the frontalis muscle. For patients whose lateral brows are already below the supraorbital rims, submuscular fascia fixation should be considered to prevent further brow ptosis.[8]

Fullness between the supratarsal crease and the brow is desirable for rejuvenated Asian male eyelids. For patients whose sub-brow region is excessively hollow, volumizing the area with fat grafting or with hyaluronic acid filler is a consideration. Fat grafting of the upper eyelid has been described elsewhere,[9] as has volumization with hyaluronic acid filler,[10] both of which can be performed simultaneously or as separate procedures. Volumization with fat grafting or filler injection may require multiple treatments, so the patient should be appropriately counseled.

Complications

The most significant potential complication of Asian male blepharoplasty is related to the strength and position of the supratarsal crease, especially for younger patients. Even a tiny difference in the appearance between the 2 eyes can

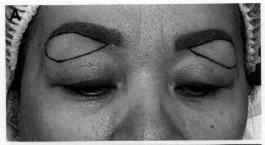

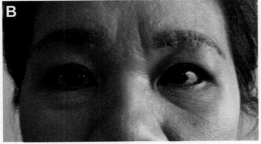

Fig. 3. Markings for sub-brow blepharoplasty. For older Asian male patients, this technique is preferred. Many patients exhibit dermatochalasis laterally more than medially, and removal of excess skin with this approach allows the surgeon to correct the lateral dermatochalasis, even past the lateral canthus, without a long supratarsal scar. The operative markings in (A) show the amount of sub-brow skin to be excised, with the widest aspect lateral to the lateral canthus. Six weeks after surgery (B) the scars are very well hidden.

be a point of scrutiny for the patient, from himself and from others. It is critical for the patient to have appropriate expectations of pretarsal swelling, especially in the immediate postoperative period. A strong high crease with excessive pretarsal show is especially undesirable, and it can occur in patients who have underlying subtle ptosis. The surgeon must be careful to evaluate ptosis in the preoperative evaluation. It is easy for the condition to become worse because of the increased weight on the levator apparatus that comes with the new double eyelid crease formation. If there is concern about uneven or undesirable appearance, revision surgery can be performed 6 months after the initial surgery.

Another complication to consider in Asian male blepharoplasty that is not as big an issue in non-Asian males is scarring, especially for patients who undergo surgery with the sub-brow approach. To minimize the appearance of the sub-brow scar, meticulous surgical technique is critical. It starts with the incision, which must be beveled to avoid transecting hair follicles, and ends with careful tension-free closure and approximation of the skin edges. If there is concern of postoperative scarring,

regular treatment with triamcinolone injections can help improve the outcome.

Asian male rhinoplasty

In recent years, we have witnessed a surge in popularity of rhinoplasty among Asian men, reflecting the growing demand for facial cosmetic procedures in both Western and Eastern societies. This article delves into the various aspects of this trend, exploring the confluence of cultural, esthetic, and anatomic factors that ultimately shape the surgical approach. In contrast with the modest esthetic goals achievable by rudimentary surgical techniques of the past, contemporary Asian male rhinoplasty aims to distill the collective elements thought to be attractive across modern industrialized cultures.

The rise in Asian male rhinoplasty appears at least partially linked to the explosion of social media and the interplay between these media dynamics and social influence.[11,12] Social media applications craft a virtual space where beauty is curated with meticulous effort and forethought. Photo editing and retouching, once the realm of beauty magazine editorials, has become available to anyone with a phone. Face filters, capable of subtle or drastic alterations, contribute to a digital realm celebrating enhanced esthetics and often idealized standards. At least in part, exposure to these images helps fuel a desire among Asian males to achieve these popularized appearances through rhinoplasty.

As mentioned, a corollary is the inescapable reach of K-pop, as its global influence has had a massive impact in redefining beauty standards for Asian males. Icons in this genre, celebrated for symmetric, refined facial features, with projected and defined noses, become aspirational benchmarks. The quest to emulate the esthetic appeal of these pop stars has likely served as a catalyst in strengthening the growing inclination among Asian men toward rhinoplasty.

Beyond individual aspirations, social pressures within Asian cultures significantly contribute to the rise of Asian male rhinoplasty. Cultural norms and workplace expectations regarding appearance, coupled with the fear of societal judgment, propel individuals toward cosmetic procedures. The intersection of cultural influences with globalized beauty standards creates a complex tapestry of motivations, indicating Asian male rhinoplasty will remain a growing segment of the population seeking rhinoplasty.

Culture in rhinoplasty

Lamentably, Asian rhinoplasty continues to be approached and performed by a subset of surgeons without adequate consideration for the unique nuances associated with each patient's ethnicity and culture; beyond intrinsic anatomic disparities, these nuances are the deeply rooted and individual esthetic preferences that make each patient unique. Asian male rhinoplasty, and rhinoplasty more broadly, cannot be approached as an algorithmic operation with a fixed set of steps that, when executed, guarantees both functional and esthetic success. Especially in contemporary society, beauty in rhinoplasty cannot be effectually defined by a collection of strict measurements or angles.

Even within the subset of Asian male rhinoplasty patients, goals and desires can vary widely based on that patient's specific background. This can be seen clearly in the differences often encountered between Eastern and Southeast Asian cultures. While sharing some similarities, they also exhibit distinct characteristics that influence their perspectives and goals of cosmetic surgery. In Eastern Asian patients such as Chinese, Japanese, and Korean, there is often a deep-rooted emphasis on modern beauty standards. Cosmetic procedures, particularly rhinoplasty, are often sought to align with these ideals. In contrast, Southeast Asian cultures, including patients from Thailand, Vietnam, and Indonesia, often desire a broader range of facial features and skin tones. Here, the goal of rhinoplasty may be more conservative when compared to Eastern patient populations.

Among the subset of Asians seeking rhinoplasty, we can make certain anatomic generalizations about the nasal dorsum. These include a smaller nasal pyramid, with shorter and often wider nasal bones leading to a deeper radix and a lower-than-ideal nasal starting point; a thinner, shorter, and weaker quadrangular septal cartilage; and wider dorsal esthetic lines.[13] This makes dorsal augmentation a frequent and crucial aspect of successful surgery. Accomplishing this augmentation in the setting of weak and often short, native nasal cartilage, with resultant poor nasal tip support, compounds the challenge of creating lasting augmentation and projection.

While historically desultory materials like ivory and jade were used for dorsal augmentation, contemporary techniques have evolved a substantial degree.[14] Surgeons now focus on minimizing complications associated with artificial implants while maximizing results using autologous grafts.

Alloplastic techniques
Despite associated risks that will be detailed in the following sections, silicone implants have maintained their presence in contemporary Asian male rhinoplasty due to their inherent simplicity and ease of placement. These implants encompass a diverse array of types, each characterized by variations in composition, shape, and size. However, they collectively share a heightened vulnerability to implant-related complications, including infection, migration, visibility, and extrusion, when contrasted with their autologous counterparts.[15]

Prior to moving forward with alloplastic augmentation rhinoplasty, patients must be thoroughly counseled not only with regards to the potential complications but also as far as the expected transition and evolution of the overlying nasal skin, which tends to attenuate, revealing the silicone implant's presence. Late changes in contour may also manifest with the development of microcalcifications on the implant surface and subsequent irregularities.

Thinning of the nasal skin can also contribute toward implant extrusion, heralded by redness, pain along the implant, and skin ulceration. Implant extrusion mandates immediate remedial measures, entailing the removal of the implant, debridement, excision of the implant capsule, and judicious administration of appropriate antibiotic therapy. In this setting, the consideration of immediate reconstruction is imprudent, as the compromised vascularity and elasticity of the skin envelope would result in suboptimal results.[16]

In an attempt to avoid implant extrusion and improve skin contour surrounding the implant, combined autologous/alloplastic techniques have been used. These techniques often involve placing a silicone implant along the nasal dorsum, with autologous cartilage grafting being used for nasal tip augmentation and support. Despite a somewhat lower risk profile, synthetic implantation (even confined to the nasal dorsum) continue to show increased rates of complications including extrusion, infection, and damage to the skin soft-tissue envelope when compared to autologous augmentation.

Autologous techniques—en bloc cartilage grafting
Recently, many surgeons are pivoting away from synthetic augmentation. This has aided in the development of advanced techniques to better utilize autologous tissues in producing a safe, long-term alternative to synthetic grafting. While various methodologies have been attempted, including dermal fat, fascia, perichondrium, bone grafting, and/or costal cartilage-costal cartilage techniques, either en bloc or diced cartilage wrapped in fascia (DCF) has emerged as the one of the

most effective options for Asian rhinoplasty—either male or female.[17–19]

The application of costal cartilage as an en bloc dorsal onlay demands a high level of surgical proficiency and experience. This technique necessitates the harvesting of a continuous, single piece of cartilage of sufficient length to span the dorsum. Furthermore, the surgeon must possess the acumen to select the appropriate segment of the rib cartilage that can withstand warping and the technical expertise to carve and chamfer the graft into a natural-appearing shape devoid of visible irregularities. Meticulous dissection to create a snug pocket capable of accommodating the dorsal onlay graft is also paramount. This serves to diminish the potential for graft migration or deviation.

However, en bloc techniques still show a propensity to deviate and any deviation of the augmentation will result in total deviation of the augmentation placed since the cartilage is, of course, en bloc. Various strategies have been explored to mitigate the risk of movement, including creating a concavity on the ventral surface of the graft, roughening the native dorsum, the deployment of K-wires, percutaneous sutures, transcutaneous sutures, and the application of tissue adhesives.

Autologous techniques—diced cartilage grafting

In an attempt to minimize the common complications and pitfalls associated with en bloc cartilage grafting (warping, need for K-wire fixation, deviation of the en bloc graft), DCF augmentation has gained popularity. Originally detailed by the works of F. Burian, Erol, Guerrerosantos, and Rollin Daniel,[20,21] cartilage is finely diced and then wrapped in temporalis fascia creating a soft, customizable augmentation graft. This avoids en bloc warping and the need for precise harvesting and carving. This technique has proven to create natural, long-lasting results with minimal complications or need for revision of the dorsal augmentation.

More recently, tissue adhesives have been use to bind the diced cartilage, forming the so-called diced cartilage glue graft (DCGG). [17,22] This removes the need of fascia harvest, relieves the burden of creating a fascial sheath, and shortens operative times. Because of this, using fibrin glue to create a solid augmentation graft has grown in prevalence. This does not mean DCGG is without specific risks. Attention to finely dicing the cartilage to avoid a cobblestone appearance of the dorsal skin is required. Since the diced cartilage is placed immediate deep to the nasal soft tissue envelope, the risk of tissue irregularities is higher when compared to DCF techniques. Postoperative inflammation can also be increased due to the presence of tissue adhesives. Finally, warping or breakdown of the augmentation can occur if the graft is not created with sufficient diced cartilage and adhesive.

Alar Base Modification Techniques

The alar base plays a significant role in the overall esthetic of the nose. This includes the width of the alar base and contour of the ala itself. In Asian male rhinoplasty, where alar base modification is a frequent request, judicious modification is advised, and avoidance of over resection is a must.

A common concern in Asian rhinoplasty is addressing excessive alar flaring. This is often modified through techniques that involve excising a small portion of the ala, performed in a V-shaped or wedgelike manner. The incision is placed either at the alar-facial junction or immediately above the alar-facial junction. This reduction narrows the alar base by reducing the degree of alar flare, creating a more refined nostril contour. Again, judicious resection is advised.

For patients with a wide nasal base with increased nasal sill width, alar base narrowing techniques with specific sill reduction are used to reduce the distance between the 2 alar bases. While alar base–binding sutures have been used in the past, more recently, sill narrowing is achieved by excising a portion of the nasal sill directly, thereby decreasing the nasal width. Alar base narrowing can be performed in conjunction with alar flare reduction to improve the alar base width and shape (**Figs. 4** and **5**).

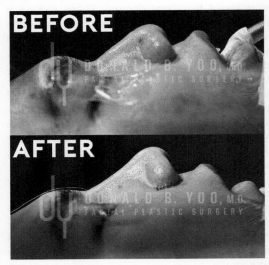

Fig. 4. The combination of unified tip grafts with alar base modification utilizing Weir and sill incisions to increase tip definition while reducing the width, thickness, and flare of the ala. (Image Courtesy Donald B. Yoo, MD.)

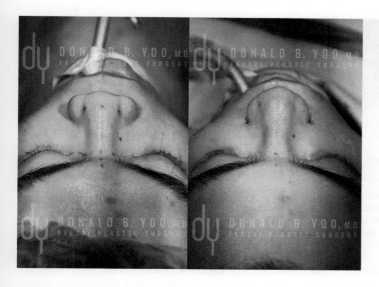

Fig. 5. Top-down intraoperative view demonstrating the significant reshaping effected by unified tip grafting and alar base modification with combined Weir and sill incisions. (Image Courtesy Donald B. Yoo, MD.)

The decision to perform alar base modification in Asian rhinoplasty should be based on careful consideration of the patient's unique facial anatomy, esthetic goals, and cultural factors. Once a surgical plan is agreed upon, computer morphed images should be used to aid in the amount of modification performed. Finally, when modifying the alar base, err on the side of caution. Always be willing to perform an additional resection for further narrowing at a later date to avoid over resection at the time of surgery (**Fig. 6**).

Nasal tip esthetics

Especially during Asian male rhinoplasty, tip definition cannot be created simply by removing excess tissue and volume from the tip complex, as the thickness and sebaceous quality of the skin envelope will obscure the underlying shape of the nasal framework and the intrinsic lack of strength in the nasal framework will preclude attempts at forming durable tip projection and esthetics without appropriate structural reinforcement. In thin-skinned patients with strong lower lateral cartilages, suture techniques with or without excision of cartilage and subcutaneous fat may provide sufficient refinement along the nasal tip complex. However, these same maneuvers would fail to produce any refinement of the supra-alar groove, lateral tip, or supratip in the overwhelming majority of Asian male patients.

For Asian male rhinoplasty, approaches that add structure to the framework of the nose while

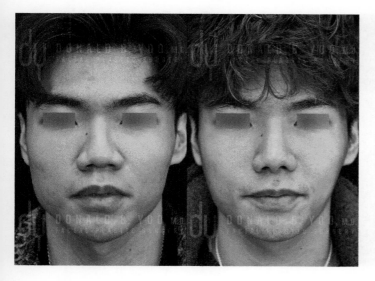

Fig. 6. Postoperative view after male Asian rhinoplasty with rib cartilage, diced cartilage wrapped in fascia (DCF), and alar base modification. (Image Courtesy Donald B. Yoo, MD.)

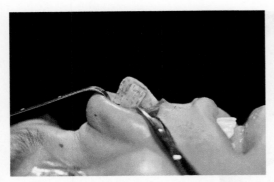

Fig. 7. Extended spreader grafts reinforcing the dorsal septum and supporting a robust septal extension graft and spacer graft (fashioned from autologous costal cartilage) in-line with the caudal septum.

preserving and re-orienting the existing nasal cartilage provide the most durable and esthetically successful results. While a minority of surgeons cling to suboptimal techniques reliant on alloplastic or homoplastic implants, most contemporary surgeons have embraced the use of autologous costal cartilage, ear cartilage, and/or temporalis fascia to supplement cartilage available in the nose. The unified tip technique is the preferred approach of the senior author, as it addresses the infratip-to-columellar ratio, infratip break, tip volume, supra-alar and lateral tip, and supratip while providing a smooth, natural-appearing contour and maximal structural symmetry for permanent results.

The basis of the unified tip theory is the premise that the septum provides the foundation of a more projected and defined nose in male Asian rhinoplasty. Extended spreader grafts and a septal extension graft serve as force multipliers to allow

for an even stronger foundation than the innate septum to provide a platform to secure the lower lateral cartilages in a tensioned and more refined orientation, while enhancing the ratio between the columella and infratip and reducing volume along the lateral tip (**Fig. 7**). Upon establishing a triangulated base, the tip and ala may further be modified and enhanced by recreating the nasal tip topography using integrated alar rim and tip grafts (**Figs. 8** and **9**). In this way, nasal tip projection and rotation may be manipulated independently of the size and shape of the lower lateral cartilages, thereby obviating the reliance on tradrational tip support mechanisms (**Fig. 10**).[23–25]

Operative technique

Before surgery, the patient is marked while seated in the preoperative holding area. Key markings include the nasal starting point, any dorsal convexity, desired supratip break, and various facial landmarks. For costal cartilage harvest, the xiphoid and inframammary crease are marked. The nose is opened with care taken to create a precise dorsal picket for the placement of the dorsal augmentation graft. DCF is typically necessary in Asian rhinoplasty for dorsal augmentation, as septal cartilage alone is usually insufficient.

Preserving ≥15 mm of dorsal and caudal struts in Asian patients is recommended to maintain structural integrity. The platform created by the convergence of upper lateral cartilages may require modification for a smoother contour. Careful attention is required for supratip break projection and angle, especially in cases of increased tip projection and nasal lengthening. This often requires extended spreader graft placement and septal extension graft placement.

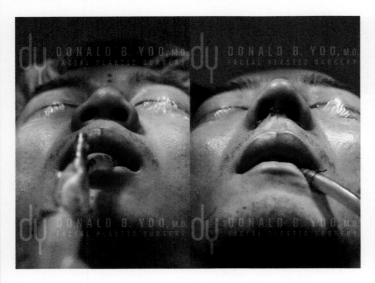

Fig. 8. Tip and alar reshaping using unified tip grafts and sill incisions to define the tip, reduce the width and flare of the ala, and to narrow the nostrils. (Image Courtesy Donald B. Yoo, MD.)

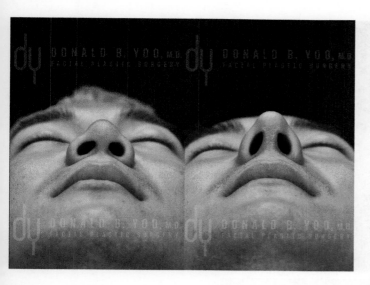

Fig. 9. Postoperative view of tip and alar reshaping using unified tip grafts and sill incisions to define the tip, reduce the width and flare of the ala, and to narrow the nostrils. Proper design, placement, and execution of incisions create virtually imperceptible scars. (Image Courtesy Donald B. Yoo, MD.)

Osteotomies may be performed when the nasal bones remain excessively wide or deviated. In cases of a dorsal hump deformity, augmentation is typically provided by removing the contributing bone and cartilage. Once this is accomplished, the native nasal dorsum must be checked for any irregularities or asymmetries which could translate to contour irregularities after the augmentation graft is placed. When the hump is substantial, DCF may be designed to contain diced cartilage above the hump, providing a smooth transition with fascia below it. Auricular conchal cartilage may be harvested for DCF in cases requiring mild to moderate augmentation (**Fig. 11**).

Costal cartilage is often required in cases demanding moderate to significant augmentation based on the sheer volume of cartilage required. Cartilage is diced into fine particles, ensuring a smooth, uniform contour, and is then inserted into a cylindrical sheath. Deep temporalis fascia is harvested, thinned, cut into precise dimensions, and is used as a sheath to wrap the diced cartilage for dorsal augmentation. DCF is typically performed after establishing tip projection, rotation, and length (**Fig. 12**).

Additional refinements to the DCF technique can be made for consistent and predictable results. A mattress suture is used to create a portion filled with fine, diced cartilage to augment the dorsum, with the rest of the fascia draping over the supratip and tip complex. Fenestrations are made in the graft to allow for fluid efflux, cartilage volume evaluation, and swelling resolution. Corset sutures are placed according to the patient's dorsal esthetic lines (**Fig. 13**).

Percutaneous sutures secure the DCF to the marked nasal starting point. The size, shape, and augmentation can be adjusted by redraping the skin envelope with the DCF in place, and the final shape is determined with a thermoplastic splint. The cast is shaped and solidified to achieve the desired dorsum.

After the nasal dorsum has been augmented and the nasal tip projection and rotation have been set, alar base modifications are carried out.

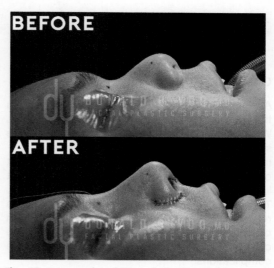

Fig. 10. Increased stability of the nasal framework provided by the addition of structural costal cartilage grafts, allowing for increased nasal tip projection and improved definition of the nasal tip and ala. (Image Courtesy Donald B. Yoo, MD.)

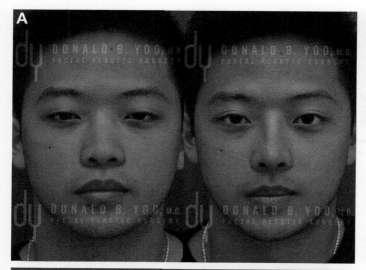

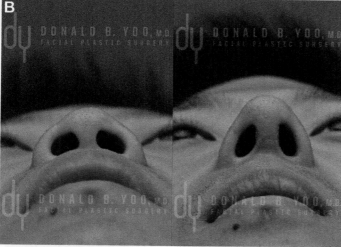

Fig. 11. (*A*) Frontal view of Asian male rhinoplasty patient who underwent open rhinoplasty with rib cartilage and DCF (diced cartilage wrapped in fascia) with unified tip grafts to improve the refinement and shape of his nasal tip complex. (*B*) Base view of Asian male rhinoplasty patient who underwent open rhinoplasty with rib cartilage and DCF (diced cartilage wrapped in fascia) with unified tip grafts to improve the refinement and shape of his nasal tip complex. (Image Courtesy Donald B. Yoo, MD.)

COMPLICATIONS

As with any surgical intervention, there is always the possibility of encountering complications. While meticulous planning and knowledge of the surgical techniques will help avoid issues, accurately identifying problems as they occur will not only aid in management but also can prevent long-term sequelae related to the occurrence. To facilitate a discussion of complications related to Asian rhinoplasty, we will begin with preoperative issues, elaborate on intraoperative concerns, and finally conclude with postoperative complications.

Preoperative Complications

Formulating a surgical plan in Asian rhinoplasty begins with a thorough assessment of the

patient's baseline anatomy and esthetic objectives. Aligning the patient's perception of beauty with the surgeon's understanding is pivotal to achieving patient satisfaction. Subjective terms

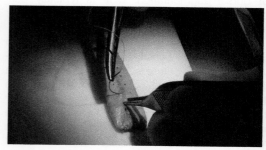

Fig. 12. Corset sutures to refine the shape of the dorsal esthetic lines.

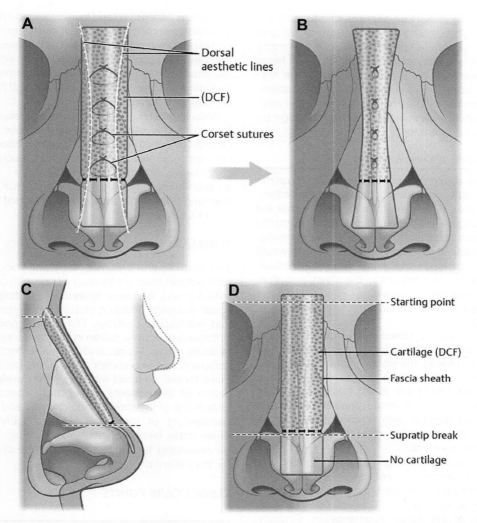

Fig. 13. (*A, B*) Proper placement of the diced cartilage wrapped in fascia (DCF) graft, extending slightly cephalad beyond the desired starting point to the anticipate future contracture, and the cephalad portion comprised of fascia without diced cartilage secured over the supratip and tip. (*C*) Refining the frontal shape of the diced cartilage fascia (DCF) graft, and subsequently the dorsum, with corset sutures by recreating the natural curvature of the dorsal esthetic lines. (*D*) With accurate placement of the corset sutures, the overall width of the DCF graft as well as the convergence and divergence of the dorsal esthetic lines can be precisely controlled. (*From* Ghavami, A., Most, S., & Cerkes, N. Global Rhinoplasty: A Multicultural Approach. Georg Thieme Verlag, 2023.)

do very little in achieving this understanding. Often patients will request things to be "improved," or to make things "better," and "cuter." One's version of cute can vary wildly depending on personal preferences. So, to create a more granular surgical plan, employing standardized imaging is an absolute necessity.

Computer morphing is also a valuable tool, allowing for interactive adjustments and visualization in collaboration with the patient. It provides insights into the desired level of augmentation, the optimal nasal starting point, the configuration of the supratip to tip transition, and the overall dimensions and contour of the nasal dorsum. Further, this will again allow avoidance of vague descriptors and instead provide actual goals with objective amounts and degrees.

During the preoperative evaluation and review of imaging, the surgeon must also educate the patient on how their specific anatomy will influence the postoperative appearance of their nose and dorsum. Discussions include factors such as the size, shape, and projection of the forehead, lips, and chin, as well as the selection of an appropriate nasal starting point and the desired configuration of the supratip-to-tip transition.

This dialog is not just about understanding the patient's goals but also about introducing any anatomic or patient-specific limitations that might affect the feasibility of certain objectives. It helps the surgeon identify suitable candidates for surgery and cases where surgery may be inadvisable. Establishing a solid esthetic framework and realistic preoperative expectations sets the stage for a successful operation.

Intraoperative Complications

The use of autologous costal cartilage in Asian rhinoplasty does carry additional associated intraoperative risk. First, there is a possibility that the costal cartilage has become calcified. While partial calcification does produce useable grafting material, complete or near-complete calcification would render the cartilage unusable. This is often associated with previous trauma to the chest, radiation, or excessive use of corsets or girdles. Age can be related but is not an absolute indicator of calcification.

During harvest of costal cartilage there is also a risk of pneumothorax. After the cartilage segment has been removed, the wound should be filled with normal saline. A Valsalva maneuver is then performed, identifying any area of air egress. If an injury is identified, immediate repair should be performed in conjunction with removal of any intrathoracic air. Postoperative chest X ray will dictate further management.

Once suitable grafting material has been obtained, a dorsal pocket must be precisely dissected to accommodate the required augmentation. Excess dissection leads to increased migration of the dorsal augmentation. Similarly, casting must be done with great care to avoid indention or shifting of the augmentation graft.

Postoperative Complications

Diced cartilage techniques for dorsal augmentation result in early postoperative edema and can mask issues with graft placement, symmetry, and overall contour of the result. Varying skin characteristics along the nasal skin envelope result in uneven swelling, which may benefit from periodic triamcinolone and 5-fluorouracil injections during recovery.

In the initial 2 months of recovery, minor graft placement and contour issues can often be addressed with gentle DCF massage before the graft solidifies. Major misplacements may require surgery. In primary Asian rhinoplasty, contour irregularities can relate to surgical technique, but these can be minimized with precise intraoperative execution. However, previous scarring and revision rhinoplasty cases may lead to unexpected irregularities and asymmetry. To help minimize asymmetric dorsal graft placement, it is important to ensure the recipient-site base is even, without bony ridges or asymmetries. Careful attending to smoothing any dorsal irregularities prior to the placement of the dorsal augmentation graft must be done.

Following full healing, minor contour issues can be managed similarly to en bloc cartilage grafts. Over-augmentation or under-augmentation is a common complication. Preoperative discussions can help mitigate this issue, but under-augmentation may require additional DCF, while over-augmentation may necessitate dorsal reduction or DCF removal.

SUMMARY

The landscape of blepharoplasty and rhinoplasty for the Asian male is intricately woven with cultural, esthetic, and anatomic nuances, reflecting a dynamic interplay between global beauty standards and individual aspirations. The surge in popularity of these procedures, driven in part by the influence of social media, K-pop, and societal expectations, underscores the complex motivations behind the quest for refined facial esthetics. With careful evaluation of the patients' goals and expectations, knowledge of the anticipated anatomy, and an understanding of the latest surgical techniques, Asian male blepharoplasty and rhinoplasty can be rewarding for the surgeon and life-changing for the patients.

CLINICS CARE POINTS

- Younger Asian male blepharoplasty patients are best served with a supratarsal approach to create or reinforce the double eyelid in a natural manner.

- Older male Asian blepharoplasty patients are best served with a sub-brow approach to improve the dermatochalasis while minimizing the degree of change in appearance.

- Adjunct procedures including medial epicanthoplasty, lateral canthoplasty, or volumization with fat or filler should be considered when appropriate.

- The nasal dorsum in many Asian patients will have a deep nasofrontal angle with wide nasal bones and low middle vault.

- The nasal septum will be short with minimal cartilage for grafting.

- Effective communication is essential in reviewing and establishing operative goals.

- DCF shaping and sizing must be customized on a patient-by-patient basis.
- If shifting of the DCF is noticed in the immediate postoperative period, applying finger pressure can be attempted to adjust the position.

DISCLOSURE

The authors have nothing to disclose.

REFERENCES

1. Lieu S, Wu WTL, Chan HH, et al. Consensus on changing trends, attitudes, and concepts of asian beauty. Aesth Plast Surg 2016;40:193–201.
2. Kwon SH, Lao WWK, Lee CH, et al. Experiences and attitudes toward aesthetic procedures in east asia: a cross-sectional survey of five geographical regions. Arch Plast Surg 2021;48(6):660–9.
3. Cho I. Principle and mechanism of double eyelid formation. Arch Plast Surg 2023;50(2):142–7.
4. Kim YJ, Lee KH, Choi HL, et al. Cosmetic lateral canthoplasty: preserving the lateral canthal angle. Arch Plast Surg 2016;43(4):316–20.
5. Baek JS, Choi YJ, Jang JW. Medial epicanthoplasty: what works and what does not. Facial Plast Surg 2020;36(5):584–91.
6. Lam SM. Aesthetic facial surgery for the asian male. Facial Plast Surg 2005;21(4):317–23.
7. Hayashi T, Fujimori R, Hirota R, et al. Usefulness of sub-eyebrow rhytidectomy. J Jpn Aesthetic Plastic Surg 2003;25:114–8.
8. Kim WJ, Kim HK, Bae TH, et al. Analysis of subbrow upper blepharoplasty by measuring the lid-to-brow distance. Arch Aesthetic Plast Surg 2019;25(2):45–51.
9. Larsson JC, Chen TY, Lao WW. Integrating fat graft with blepharoplasty to rejuvenate the asian periorbita. Plast Reconstr Surg Glob Open 2019;7(10):2365e.
10. Montes JR, Santos E, Amaral C. Eyelid and periorbital dermal fillers: products, techniques, and outcomes. Facial Plast Surg Chin North Am 2021;29(2):335–48.
11. Jang YJ, Yu MS. Rhinoplasty for the Asian nose. Facial Plast Surg 2010;26(2):93–101.
12. Kwak ES. Asian cosmetic facial surgery. Facial Plast Surg 2010;26(2):102–9.
13. Patel PN, Most SP. Concepts of facial aesthetics when considering ethnic rhinoplasty. Otolaryngol Clin North Am 2020;53(2):195–208.
14. MILLARD DR. Oriental peregrinations. Plast Reconstr Surg (1946) 1955;16(5):319–36.
15. Waldman SR. Gore-Tex for nasal augmentation. Plast Reconstr Surg 1995;96(1):228–9.
16. Wang TD. Gore-Tex nasal augmentation: a 26-year perspective. Arch Facial Plast Surg 2011;13(2):129–30.
17. Yoo SH, Jang YJ. Rib cartilage in Asian rhinoplasty: new trends. Curr Opin Otolaryngol Head Neck Surg 2019;27(4):261–6.
18. Gurley JM, Pilgram T, Perlyn CA, et al. Long-term outcome of autogenous rib graft nasal reconstruction. Plast Reconstr Surg 2001;108(7):1895–905. discussion 1906-7.
19. Menick FJ. Nasal reconstruction. Plast Reconstr Surg 2010;125(4):138e–50e.
20. Daniel RK, Calvert JW. Diced cartilage grafts in rhinoplasty surgery. Plast Reconstr Surg 2004;113(7):2156–71.
21. Guerrerosantos J, Trabanino C, Guerrerosantos F. Multifragmented cartilage wrapped with fascia in augmentation rhinoplasty. Plast Reconstr Surg 2006;117(3):804–12. discussion 813-6.
22. Yoo SH, Kim DH, Jang YJ. Dorsal augmentation using a glued diced cartilage graft fashioned with a newly developed mold in asian rhinoplasty. Plast Reconstr Surg 2022;150(4):757e–66e.
23. Hwang NH, Dhong ES. Septal extension graft in asian rhinoplasty. Facial Plast Surg Clin North Am 2018;26(3):331–41.
24. Byrd HS, Andochick S, Copit S, et al. Septal extension grafts: a method of controlling tip projection shape. Plast Reconstr Surg 1997;100(4):999–1010.
25. Ha RY, Byrd HS. Septal extension grafts revisited: 6-year experience in controlling nasal tip projection and shape. Plast Reconstr Surg 2003;112(7):1929–35.

Male Brow Lift and Blepharoplasty

Paris Jasmine Austell, MD, MBA*, Edwin Francis Williams III, MD

KEYWORDS

- Male brow lift • Male blepharoplasty • Upper blepharoplasty • Lower blepharoplasty
- Direct brow lift • Midforehead lift • Coronal brow lift • Endoscopic brow lift

KEY POINTS

- Understand key differences in male anatomy of the forehead, brow, and eyelid complexes.
- Learn age-related changes of the eyelid and brows in men.
- Summarize indications along with a history and physical examination of the male patient prior to undergoing brow lift and blepharoplasty.
- Learn surgical approaches to performing upper and lower blepharoplasty in men.
- Understand indications for and approaches to the direct, midforehead, coronal, pretrichial, and endoscopic brow lift techniques in the male patient.

INTRODUCTION

Understanding age-related changes to the eyelid and brow complex is the key to performing successful surgical correction in this region. Specifics of the male anatomy must be considered prior to performing brow lift and blepharoplasty in this patient population. For most men, rejuvenation of the eyelid and brow consists of modest correction in comparison to their female counterparts. Differences in esthetic norms and individual patient goals should be discussed before any surgical undertaking. The astute facial plastic surgeon also considers psychological factors in patient selection for any esthetic procedure. Realistic goals and understanding of surgical limitations are paramount for successful surgery.

ANATOMY
Brow

The brow is an important cosmetic landmark of the upper face. Its movement contributes to emotive expression and its shape is important for esthetic balance of the facial structure. The medial aspect lies along the alar-facial crease. Laterally, the brow rests along a diagonal line extending to the lateral canthus. Contrary to the female brow, the ideal male brow lacks a defined arch and sits in a relatively straight line on the supraorbital rim. Age-related changes to the brow in men lead to deeper furrows than their female counterparts as a result of thicker skin.[1] As will be discussed in later sections, this has implications for choosing a surgical approach.

Forehead height in the average male measured from trichion to glabella is 7 to 8 cm.[2,3] The forehead is compartmentalized into 5 subunits: the central subunit, 2 lateral temporal subunits, and the brows.[4] Centrally, the layers of the forehead are contiguous with the scalp and are composed of skin, subcutaneous tissue, galea aponeurosis, loose areolar tissue, and periosteum. The galea envelops the paired frontalis muscles, responsible for brow elevation. At the level of the brow, frontalis fibers form confluences with the brow depressors-orbicularis oculi and procerus in addition to the overlying dermis. The corrugator and depressor supercilii, also responsible for depression of the brow, lie at the glabella and insert into the overlying dermis.[4]

Laterally in the temporal region of the forehead, the skin overlies a thin layer of subcutaneous

The Williams Center for Plastic Surgery, 1072 Troy-Schenectady Road, Latham, NY 12110, USA
* Corresponding author.
E-mail address: paustel09@gmail.com

Facial Plast Surg Clin N Am 32 (2024) 383–390
https://doi.org/10.1016/j.fsc.2024.03.002
1064-7406/24/© 2024 Elsevier Inc. All rights reserved.

tissue, which lies immediately above the superficial temporal fascia (also known as the temporoparietal fascia [TPF]). The TPF fuses with the galea of the scalp superiorly and medially as well as the superficial muscular aponeurotic system at the level of the zygoma. The facial nerve rests deep to the TPF, superficial to the deep temporal fascia. The deep temporal fascia divides into superficial and deep layers to envelop the temporal fat pad, medial to which rests the temporalis muscle.

Contraction of the frontalis and brow depressors leads to rhytids seen with aging. Along with deepening of furrows, aging of the brow leads to soft-tissue laxity and descent of the brow complex. In men with brow ptosis, unconscious frontalis contraction occurs to improve visualization and causes transverse furrows.[1] Contraction of the corrugator and depressor supercilii creates vertical glabellar lines. Transverse glabellar lines arise from contraction of the procerus.

Eyelid

The eyelids serve to protect the globe from environmental exposure and assist with the distribution of tears. At rest, the upper eyelid sits 1 to 2 mm inferior to the superior limbus. The lower eyelid sits at the level of the inferior limbus. In an esthetically appealing eye, the lateral canthus rests 2 to 4 mm superior to the medial canthus. The eyelid is composed of 2 major lamellae with the anterior portion consisting of skin and orbicularis oculi (**Fig. 1**). The posterior lamella consists of septum, tarsus, and conjunctiva. Some academicians consider the septum to be a separate "middle" lamella dividing the anterior and posterior segments.[4] The orbicularis oculi is classified into palpebral (pretarsal and preseptal) and orbital segments. The palpebral portion rests anterior to the tarsal plates and septum and is responsible for blinking. The orbital portion lies anterior to the orbital rim and is involved in forceful eye closure.

The septum is composed of connective tissue and serves as an important barrier to infection as well as an attachment for retractors of the lids. It also delineates fat compartments within the upper and lower eyelids. In the upper lid, the retroorbital fat lies posterior to the orbicularis oculi and anterior to the septum. The sub-orbicularis oculi fat (SOOF) resides in an analogous position in the lower lid. The main upper-lid retractor, the levator aponeurosis, attaches to the septum at the lid crease. In the lower lid, the septum inserts into the analogous capsulopalpebral fascia.

Within the orbit are separate fat compartments that are commonly removed in blepharoplasty.

The upper lid contains medial and central fat pads separated by the trochlea. The lateral aspect of the upper lid is occupied by the lacrimal gland. In the lower lid, fat is compartmentalized into medial, central, and lateral pockets. The inferior oblique muscle delineates the medial and central fat pads. Of note, the medial fat pad is more fibrous and paler in appearance. The arcuate expansion creates a partition between the central and lateral fat pads.

Aging of the upper eyelid leads to excess skin, or dermatochalasis, and is the target of upper blepharoplasty. In the lower eyelid, the orbital septum weakens over time and causes pseudo-herniation of the orbital fat pads. Additionally, descent of the SOOF leads to tear trough deformity and may also cause a hollowed appearance.[4]

HISTORY AND EXAMINATION

It is imperative to obtain an extensive ocular history prior to performing blepharoplasty. Conditions including dry eye, autoimmune disease (Grave's, Sjogren's, and so forth), and glaucoma are amongst a long list of disorders that may preclude cosmetic blepharoplasty.[5,6] A test of visual acuity should be conducted by the surgeon or an ophthalmologist. Schirmer's test may be used to determine the degree of dry eye, if present.[6] Lower lid laxity should be assessed with a lid distraction test. If the lid does not instantly return to anatomic position, abnormal laxity should be suspected. A distance of greater than 6 mm between the lid and cornea with distraction is also indicative of pathologic laxity. Midface aging and anatomy are also important in determining candidacy for lower blepharoplasty. A negative vector increases the risk for postoperative lid malposition and poor cosmesis if corrective adjunctive procedures are not performed.[7] The degree of upper lid skin laxity should be determined in order to more accurately assess the cosmetic outcome. In downward gaze, the distance from the upper eyelid margin to the lid crease should be 7 to 8 mm in men (in women, 8–10 mm is normal). It is prudent to assess levator function prior to blepharoplasty. When the frontalis is at rest, normal excursion of the upper lid margin from downward to upward gaze is 12 to 15 mm. Excursion less than 12 mm may be indicative of ptosis. The marginal reflex distance (MRD) measures interpalpebral distance and should also be noted to assess the need for ptosis repair. The MRD-1 is the distance between the center of the pupillary light reflex and the upper eyelid margin in primary gaze and is normally 4 to 5 mm. MRD-2 describes the distance from the lower lid margin to the corneal light reflex and is 5 mm in a normal

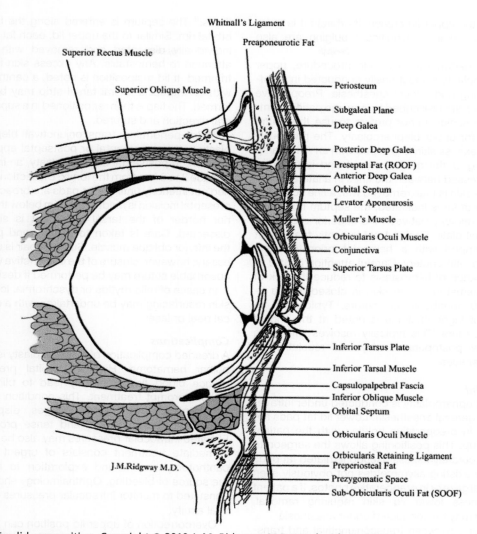

Fig. 1. Eye lid composition. Copyright © 2010 J. M. Ridgway, M.D. Used with permission.

patient. Taken together, the palpebral opening should be 9 to 10 mm. Ptosis is suspected when MRD-1 is less than the norm and may indicate levator aponeurosis dehiscence.

Brow position is important to assess prior to performing both brow lift and blepharoplasty. At rest, the male brow should sit at the level of the supraorbital rim. Many patients with brow ptosis activate their frontalis at rest to combat brow depression. To most accurately assess static brow position, patients are asked to forcefully close their eyes. Upon lid opening, the brow position is assessed. A combination of a ptotic lid and brow may be addressed in the same procedure, beginning with correction of the brow position. The degree of rhytids is assessed to assist with determination of surgical approach. Of equal importance is noting the forehead height and shape in addition to hair quality.

The esthetics of the brow including its shape and symmetry should also be noted.

SURGICAL APPROACHES
Blepharoplasty

Upper lid
The patient is examined in preoperative holding in the upright position. A surgical marking pen is used to define the supratarsal crease. It is prudent to place the brow in its anatomically correct position prior to marking the lid crease. The incision begins just lateral to the medial caruncle and extends to the lateral orbital rim. Skin is grasped until 1 to 3 mm of the orbit is exposed and the superior extent of dissection is marked at the medial limbus, pupillary line, and lateral limbus. Care is taken to leave at least 10 mm of skin from the

brow to the upper lid crease. If orbital fat is to be removed, areas of significant bulging are also marked.

When performed as a sole procedure, upper blepharoplasty is most easily conducted in an office setting under local anesthesia. Preoperative anxiolytics are prescribed to increase patient comfort. The senior author prefers to use the clamp method for upper blepharoplasty. The previously marked excess skin is grasped with an Allis clamp beginning at the medial aspect and is progressively pressed between the tines in a lateral direction. The skin is then removed with a fine scissor. If excision of fat is indicated, the septum is sharply entered midway between the superior orbital rim and tarsal plate. Each fat pat is gently teased out and clamped with a hemostat prior to being removed with cautery. Careful attention is paid to maintenance of hemostasis to reduce the risk of orbital hematoma. The skin is closed with a 6-0 or 7-0 nonabsorbable suture. Typically, 1 to 2 mm of lagophthalmos is noted at the end of the procedure. This typically resolves within the first few postoperative days as resolution of edema ensues.

Lower lid

Lower blepharoplasty is conducted under intravenous or general anesthesia. Lower lid fat pads are marked in preoperative holding with the patient looking up. This positioning allows the surgeon to most accurately assess pseudoherniated fat pads and any existing asymmetries not obviously seen in neutral gaze or in preoperative photos. If a patient has excess lower lid skin requiring removal, marking may be conducted under anesthesia.

Deciding between transconjunctival and transcutaneous approaches is dependent upon several individual patient factors. Young patients with minimal skin changes and notable fat pad pseudoherniation are best treated with a transconjunctival approach. Elderly patients or those with notable excess skin may benefit from a transcutaneous blepharoplasty. Attention must be paid to preexisting lid malposition (ectropion, entropion, and so forth), and any existing abnormalities should be corrected at the time of surgery.

If skin excision is indicated, the incision is placed 1.5 to 2 mm below the lash line. Medially, the incision begins just lateral to the inferior punctum and is carried out laterally to the orbital rim. When performed in conjunction with upper blepharoplasty, the incision is placed at least 5 to 8 mm from the upper lid incision. A skin-only flap is elevated over the pretarsal orbicularis oculi. The flap is converted to a skin-muscle flap over the septum with careful separation of the pretarsal and preseptal muscle

fibers.[8] The septum is entered along the inferior orbital rim. Similar to the upper lid, each fat pad is individually dissected and removed with great attention to hemostasis. Any excess skin is then trimmed. If lid malposition is noted, a canthopexy with or without a lateral tarsal strip may be performed. The flap is then repositioned in a superolateral direction and sutured.

When performing transconjunctival blepharoplasty, either a preseptal or postseptal approach is taken. In postseptal blepharoplasty, an incision is made 2 to 3 mm from the fornix. Dissection is carried out inferiorly until the fat pads are broached. A preseptal incision is made 1 to 2 mm below the inferior border of the tarsal plate. Fat is similarly dissected. Care is taken to identify and protect the inferior oblique muscle. Suture repair is unnecessary; however, closure of the conjunctiva with an absorbable suture may be performed if desired.

In cases of mild rhytids or dyschromia, lower lid skin resurfacing may be undertaken with a chemical peel or laser.

Complications

A dreaded complication of blepharoplasty is retrobulbar hematoma. High intraorbital pressures reduce blood flow and may lead to blindness without prompt treatment. This condition should be suspected with visual changes, disproportionate increases in pain, and tense proptosis. Elevated intraocular pressures may also be noted. Immediate treatment consists of urgent lateral canthotomy and wound exploration to identify the source of bleeding. Ophthalmology should be consulted to monitor intraocular pressures and visual acuity.

Overcorrection of upper lid position can lead to incomplete closure of the lid, or lagophthalmos. Patients may develop exposure keratitis as a result. This condition is best remedied with skin grafts harvested from the pre-auricular or post-auricular region and placed at the upper lid crease.[9] Ectropion may also result as a complication of lower lid blepharoplasty. It is typically corrected with a lateral tarsal strip procedure. In severe cases, a skin graft may be required.[9]

Brow

A multitude of surgical approaches exists for browplasty. As previously noted, anatomic considerations are particularly important for male patients including the position of the hairline and the presence of rhytids, along with forehead shape and prominence. Studies have shown no statistical difference in postoperative outcomes between different techniques.[10] Individual differences among patients and surgeon preference should be taken into consideration when choosing a surgical approach.

Direct approach

The direct brow lifting technique is the simplest, most predictable approach to brow lift as it targets the immediate area of concern.[11] It is easily performed in the office under local anesthesia. However, this approach leaves a conspicuous scar which must be taken into consideration during preoperative counseling. Direct brow lifts are an excellent option for males with balding, severe brow asymmetry, a lack of concern regarding scar appearance, and the absence of deep forehead rhytids. It is important to discuss goals of brow placement and incision length in the preoperative setting. For example, if a patient desires only lateral brow elevation, a limited incision may be placed just above the lateral aspect.

An incision is marked immediately above the most cephalically positioned brow hairs. The brow is then digitally moved to mimic the desired brow position and this is marked as the superior limb of the incision. Local anesthesia is infiltrated and the incision is undertaken with a no.15 blade. Medially, the incision is carried superficial to the frontalis muscle. Laterally, only skin is incised to avoid injury to the temporal branch of the facial nerve. If brow paralysis is noted on preoperative examination, one may elect to remove a small ellipse of frontalis muscle. The skin is then sharply excised and hemostasis achieved. The wound is closed in 2 layers with braided, absorbable, deep-dermal sutures, and nonabsorbable skin sutures.

Indirect approach

The indirect, or midforehead, approach is appropriate for male patients with existing deep rhytids. The procedure may be performed under local anesthesia with consideration of preoperative anxiolytics. This approach may leave a visible scar, which can be particularly prominent in males with thick, sebaceous skin (**Fig. 2**). An incision is marked within an existing forehead crease. When both brows are corrected, a single long incision may be made in 1 crease or 2 incisions staggered in separate creases. The incision is carried out similarly to the direct approach. Dissection is performed superficial to the frontalis muscle down to the supraorbital rim. The brow is then suspended in the desired position and secured to the frontalis with a braided, absorbable suture. The skin is closed with a nonabsorbable suture.

Coronal approach

The coronal approach is used in patients who have a low hairline with significant brow ptosis. For several years, it was the gold standard approach given its wide dissection plane which allows for correction of all aspects of forehead and brow position. The coronal lift does require a lengthy incision, which is a relative contraindication in the balding patient and may be visible in a patient with hair when wet. Additionally, patients may experience prolonged postoperative hypesthesia due to extensive dissection.[12] Intravenous or general anesthesia is typically indicated for this approach.

The incision is marked from ear to ear 4 to 6 cm posterior to the hairline. Incision is made until the galea is encountered. Dissection is performed in the subgaleal plane and the cavity is widely elevated to release the brow at the arcus marginalis and conjoint tendons. Excess skin is removed and the incision is closed in 2 layers with braided, absorbable, deep-dermal sutures, and surgical clips.

Pretrichial approach

A pretrichial brow lift is ideal for the patient with a high hairline, as it reduces vertical forehead height.[13] This approach does result in a visible scar along the hairline and similar to the coronal approach, it may lead to significant postoperative hypesthesia. Alopecia is an additional possible complication with the pretrichial approach. Patients are best treated with intravenous or general anesthesia.

An incision is marked at the hairline above the root of the helix and is carried immediately anterior to the hairline. The incision is intentionally made irregular to improve scar appearance. The brow is then released and secured similarly to the coronal brow lift approach.

Endoscopic approach

The endoscopic approach is ideal for patients who do not require change in forehead height (**Fig. 3**). Though the hairline can be raised, this approach allows modifications to be individualized to each patient. The senior author most frequently performs brow lifts via this approach under direct visualization without the use of endoscopes. This technique allows the surgeon to safely conduct a more efficient and straightforward procedure without increased morbidity. When cameras are used, patients with significant frontal bossae are not ideal candidates given inadequate visualization. Temporary shock hair loss may occur postoperatively. Either intravenous or general anesthesia is indicated for the endoscopic approach.

The senior author uses 4 incisions for this approach. Two paramedian incisions are marked vertically approximately 5 mm posterior to the hairline at the highest desired point of brow

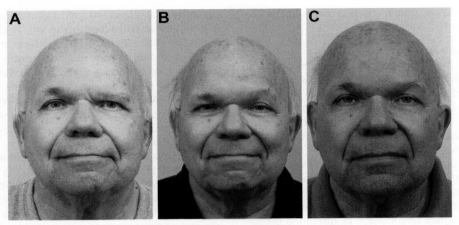

Fig. 2. (*A*) A 74-year-old male with unilateral brow asymmetry after parotidectomy. (*B*) One month after midforehead brow lift. (*C*) Seven months after midforehead brow lift with notably improved scar appearance.

elevation and are 2 to 3 cm in length.[14,15] The temporal incisions are made 2 cm posterior to the hairline and are 3 to 4 cm in length.[14] A no.15 blade is used to make the paramedian incisions until bone is visualized. Periosteal elevators are used to release the brow in a subperiosteal plane. If endoscopes are used, dissection is paused 2 cm superior to the supraorbital rim at which point cameras are introduced to clearly visualize the supraorbital neurovascular bundle. The senior author prefers gentle, blunt dissection in the region of the neurovascular bundle and has not experienced neuropraxia or significant bleeding with this technique.

The senior author cautions against corrugator and procerus resection to reduce the risk of medial brow widening and excessive elevation in this region. The temporal incisions are made until the TPF is encountered. The brow is bluntly released to the level of the lateral canthus. Care is taken not to perform complete release in this region to avoid changing the shape of the eye. If endoscopes are used, they are introduced when the conjoint tendon is encountered to avoid injury to the temporal branch of the facial nerve. The sentinel vein may be visualized and cautery is avoided in this region to reduce the risk of facial

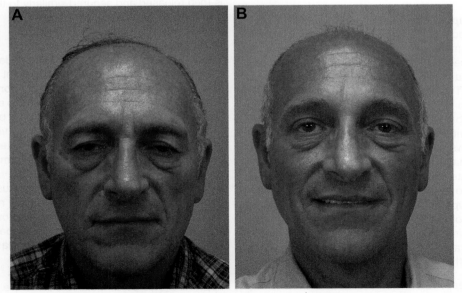

Fig. 3. (*A*) A 62-year-old male with brow ptosis and bilateral dermatochalasis. (*B*) Well-healed after endoscopic brow lift and bilateral upper blepharoplasty.

nerve injury. If cautery is necessary, a bipolar device is used with caution. The senior author prefers gentle, blunt dissection in this region under direct visualization. Bone tunnels are then drilled (accessed through paramedian incisions) and the brow is secured with a 2-0 polyglactin (Vicryl, Ethicon) suture. The temporal portion of the brow is secured to temporalis fascia and muscle with a 2-0 polyglactin suture, taking care to avoid strangulation of the muscle which may cause increased postoperative pain and trismus. Although out of the scope of this article, it is noted that midface ptosis may be addressed via this approach through temporal incisions. The incisions are then closed with braided, deep-dermal sutures, and surgical clips.

Temporal and transblepharoplasty lift

Temporal and transblepharoplasty brow lifts are indicated for lateral brow ptosis. The temporal brow lift is performed through incisions posterior to the hairline in the temporal region similar to the endoscopic approach. If a patient is undergoing upper blepharoplasty, a concomitant brow lift may be performed via the blepharoplasty incision. The senior author prefers to use these techniques in women, as it feminizes the face and is only briefly mentioned here for completeness.

Complications

Typical complications of brow lifting are similar to other surgical procedures (bleeding, scar, poor wound healing, and so forth). Hematoma requiring surgical evacuation is rare. Excessive bleeding is avoided with attention paid to hemostasis throughout the procedure. Careful dissection in the region of the superficial temporal vessels and sentinel vein reduces intraoperative and postoperative bleeding risk. A standard facelift dressing is applied and maintained for 24 hours after the procedure. Facial nerve paralysis is avoided with blunt dissection lateral to the superficial layer of the deep temporal fascia.[12] Patients should be counseled on the possibility of postoperative hypesthesia, seen most commonly with coronal and pretrichial approaches. Temporary and permanent hair losses are also discussed in preoperative counseling. Beveling of the incision allows for hair growth through scar and decreases the risk of hair loss.[12] Brow asymmetry may also occur. Pre-existing asymmetries are noted and discussed with the patient in preoperative counseling. The risk of iatrogenic asymmetry is reduced with careful attention to symmetric skin excision and suspension and full release of the arcus marginalis and conjoint tendons.[12] If asymmetry is a result of excessive elevation, release and resuspension in a more inferior

position is performed. Resection of the corrugators and procerus muscles may widen and excessively elevate the medial brow leading to an unnatural appearance.

SUMMARY

Knowledge of male anatomy is the key to performing brow lift and blepharoplasty in this population. Variations in skin thickness, brow and eyelid position, and individual patient esthetics must all be taken into consideration prior to performing these procedures. Extensive preoperative counseling regarding risks and limitations and discussion of patient goals are imperative to achieving optimal outcomes.

CLINICS CARE POINTS

- Performing brow lift and blepharoplasty in the male patient requires understanding of specific anatomic differences.
- Obtaining a thorough past medical history is essential to proper patient selection prior to blepharoplasty.
- Pre-existing lid laxity should be noted and corrected if present during male blepharoplasty.
- Skin thickness, presence of rhytids, hairline position, and patient preference on scar positioning and brow height should all be noted prior to brow lift in the male patient.

DISCLOSURE

The authors have nothing to disclose.

REFERENCES

1. Warren RJ. Upper Blepharoplasty and Brow Rejuvenation in Men. Clin Plast Surg 2022;49(2):197–212.
2. Kite A, Lucas VS. Hair transplant: a basic review. Plast Surg Nurs 2015;35(2):66–8.
3. Salinas CA, Liu A, Sharaf BA. Analysis of Hairline and Forehead Sexual Dimorphic Aesthetics in 60 Celebrities Using Artificial Intelligence. Plast Reconstr Surg Glob Open 2023;11(7):e5107. https://doi.org/10.1097/GOX.0000000000005107.
4. Ridgway JM, Larrabee WF. Anatomy for blepharoplasty and brow-lift. Facial Plast Surg 2010;26(3):177–85.
5. Patel BC, Malhotra R. Upper Eyelid Blepharoplasty. In: StatPearls. Treasure Island (FL): StatPearls Publishing; 2023.

6. Rees TD, Jelks GW. Blepharoplasty and the dry eye syndrome: guidelines for surgery? Plast Reconstr Surg 1981;68(2):249–52.

7. Sobti M, Joshi N. Lower Eyelid Blepharoplasty: Minimizing Complications and Correction of Lower Eyelid Malposition. Facial Plast Surg 2023;39(1): 28–46.

8. Massiha H. Combined Skin and Skin-Muscle Flap Technique in Lower Blepharoplasty: A 10-Year Experience. Ann Plast Surg 1990;25(6):467–76.

9. Oestreicher J, Mehta S. Complications of blepharoplasty: prevention and management. Plast Surg Int 2012;2012:252368. https://doi.org/10.1155/2012/25 2368.

10. Puig CM, LaFerriere KA. A Retrospective Comparison of Open and Endoscopic Brow-Lifts. Arch Facial Plast 2002;4(4):221–5.

11. Perry JD, Hwang CJ. Direct Browlift. Clin Plast Surg 2022;49(3):409–14.

12. Lighthall JG, Wang TD. Complications of forehead lift. Facial Plast Surg Clin North Am 2013;21(4): 619–24.

13. Dunn T, Hohman MH. Pretrichial Brow Lift. In: StatPearls. Treasure Island (FL): StatPearls Publishing; 2023. Available at: https://www.ncbi.nlm.nih.gov/books/NBK570632/.

14. Lam SM, Chang EW, Rhee JS, et al. Perspective: rejuvenation of the periocular region: a unified approach to the eyebrow, midface, and eyelid complex. Ophthalmic Plast Reconstr Surg 2004;20(1):1–9.

15. Perenack JD. The Endoscopic Brow Lift. Atlas Oral Maxillofac Surg Clin North Am 2016;24(2):165–73.

Fat Grafting the Male Face

Emily C. Deane, MD, FRCSC, MSc[a], Anni Wong, MD, MS[a], Jason D. Bloom, MD[b,c],*

KEYWORDS

- Fat grafting • Facial plastic surgery • Male gender • Facial augmentation • Facial rejuvenation
- Injectable filler

KEY POINTS

- The facial plastic surgeon must have a firm understanding of skeletal and soft tissue anatomic divergences, as well as unique biologic and histologic features, relating to each gender.
- Fat grafting can be used for structural enhancement of male facial features that may wane with aging, namely the mandible, chin, brow and midface. It can improve skin quality in areas like the neck.
- Targeted augmentation with fat should be performed carefully to avoid feminizing the face.
- Males are at increased risk for bruising and bleeding from facial cosmetic procedures, including fat grafting.

 Video content accompanies this article at http://www.facialplastic.theclinics.com.

BACKGROUND

During recent decades, the proportion of men interested in aesthetic treatments has progressively increased. According to the 2020 American Society of Aesthetic Plastic Surgery Report, male patients make up 8% of aesthetic patients, up to 75% of those undergoing minimally-invasive procedures.[1] In a survey of over 14,000 adults, there were clear gender-related differences in cosmetic concerns and motivations,[2] highlighting the importance of evaluating male patients with a different lens. Two of the top five most common concerns of respondents were dark circles or under eye hollowing, and lack of volume or definition in the cheeks.[2] Many male patients express a desire to address their "tired" appearance, to maintain their masculinity while avoiding stigmata of a cosmetic intervention.

Autologous fat grafting is a minimally-invasive technique to restore or establish facial volume and structure, often used in combination with other treatments for facial rejuvenation. Adipose tissue is readily available, easy to harvest and inexpensive with little donor-site morbidity. Fat is softer and more compressible than alloplastic filler and is frequently injected in a multilayered fashion to provide panfacial volumization. Unlike other injectable materials, adipose tissue does not trigger an immunologic response that could lead to rejection.

There are a number of articles describing injectable techniques for the male face,[3–7] but few specifically address autologous facial fat grafting for men.[8] Previous studies have shown that male patients tend to favor interventions requiring the fewest number of repeat visits, which may make fat grafting a more attractive option than injectable fillers.[3] As with many facial plastic surgical interventions, care must be taken when performing autologous fat grafting for men, as it is possible to unintentionally feminize the region being treated. Although autologous fat grafting is also used for reconstructive[9] and gender-affirming

[a] Facial Plastic & Reconstructive Surgery, Department of Otolaryngology Head & Neck Surgery, University of Pennsylvania, 3737 Market Street, Suite 302, Philadelphia, PA 19104, USA; [b] Facial Plastic & Reconstructive Surgery, Department of Otolaryngology Head & Neck Surgery, University of Pennsylvania, Philadelphia, PA, USA; [c] Bloom Facial Plastic Surgery, Two Town Place, Suite 110, Bryn Mawr, PA 19010, USA
* Corresponding author. Bloom Facial Plastic Surgery, Two Town Place, Suite 110, Bryn Mawr, PA 19010.
E-mail address: drjbloom@bloomfps.com

Facial Plast Surg Clin N Am 32 (2024) 391–398
https://doi.org/10.1016/j.fsc.2024.03.003
1064-7406/24/© 2024 Elsevier Inc. All rights reserved.

procedures, this review will focus on its use for aging face as a stand-alone or adjunctive procedure.

The facial plastic surgeon must have a firm understanding of skeletal and soft-tissue anatomic divergences, as well as unique biologic and histologic features, relating to each gender. Male facial skin is 30 to 175 microns thicker than that of females, is more elastic and vascular, and has relatively less subcutaneous fat.[10] Males have a higher density of terminal-hair follicular units and dermal adnexal structures under the influence of testosterone. Conversely, estrogen contributes to the greater quantity of subcutaneous fat, a smoother female facial contour and softer appearance of muscular contraction during mimetic movements.[11] Interestingly, distinct regional histocytologic differences have been seen in facial adipose compartments, some which may also be affected by sex.[12]

FACIAL AGING IN MEN

There are many developmental sexual dimorphisms of the human face,[13] and thereby differences in the manner in which they age. Men typically have a larger skull, squarer face with an angular, wider and larger mandible. Men are more equally balanced in their upper and lower facial proportions, compared to the tapering craniofacial anatomy of women.[14] For both sexes, posterior displacement of the maxilla, enlargement of the orbital and pyriform apertures, increased gonial angle with decreased size of the bony mandible, all occur with aging.[15] Senile bone loss occurs linearly in men compared to the more precipitous bone loss experienced by women after menopause, although this has been less well characterized in facial aging than in other parts of the bony skeleton.[16]

The underlying processes of facial skin aging that result from endogenous (eg, genetic) or exogenous (eg, UV exposure) are similar in men and women. Predisposing social factors including smoking or occupational sun exposure, however, have been historically more common for men and may underlie the observed rapid-onset changes in skin quality. Male rhytids tend to appear as prominent, deeper lines rather than fine lines seen in women[4] and they develop earlier. The male wrinkle pattern is thought to be due to differences in facial muscle tone, skin thickness and adnexal structures and lack of significant subcutaneous fat.[14,17]

In the past, gravity was understood to underlie most deeper soft-tissue aging changes, and hence early facial rejuvenation efforts relied primarily on lifting and tightening of these tissues.

More recently, there has been a growing body of evidence that volumetric changes of facial adipose play a more important role.[12,18–20] It is theorized that as deeper fat compartments deflate, more superficial compartments not only lose volume but also experience a weakening of their support and anatomically become ptotic. Age-related depletion of the facial fat pads result in decreased facial projection, hollowing and sagging of overlying skin due to relative excess.[18] Similar to bone loss, steady atrophy of facial soft tissue occurs in men as opposed to the rapid decline found in perimenopausal women.

PATIENT SELECTION, ASSESSMENT & TREATMENT PLANNING

A thorough patient history, including medications, particularly anticoagulant or anti-platelet agents, history of poor wound healing or hypertrophic scars/keloids, history of cold sores and prior cosmetic procedures should be performed. Physical examination should focus on delineating asymmetries of the face, temporal and periorbital hollowing, midface width and malar fat pad descent, jaw contour deficiencies and the presence of jowling. Very thin patients are poor candidates for fat grafting as harvest can lead to unacceptable cosmetic changes of the donor site. It is also important to assess for previous surgical scars at potential donor sites, as these may hinder one's ability to harvest fat adequately. Patients with poor endovascular health may be predisposed to complications.

The decision to perform autologous fat grafting under local versus general anesthesia depends on patient tolerance, surgeon preference and the performance of concurrent procedures. Some authors recommend anticipatory treatment with neurotoxin, for instance in the forehead and glabella, to diminish muscle movement and improve graft survival.[21]

AUTOLOGOUS FAT HARVEST, PROCESSING & TRANSFER TECHNIQUES
Harvest Sites & Instruments

Donor site selection is based on the amount of fat required, surgeon preference and occasionally patient preference. The most common donor sites include the lower abdomen, flank and inner thigh followed by the knee and buttocks.[21,22] Peripheral fat distribution varies between sexes; men tend to have less fat in the inner thigh area which may dictate a different practice pattern for preferred donor locations.

Donor site preparation may include infiltration of local anesthetic or tumescent solution, depending on surgeon preference; research regarding the most cell-protective solution for liposuction is still ongoing.[23]

A variety of fat harvesting cannulas are commercially available and selection depends on volume of fat to be collected. Fat grafting for facial rejuvenation is considered 'small-volume' when compared to other sites (ie, <100 cc). Lipoharvest cannulas differ primarily in diameter and number of holes; both variables are suggested to influence the success of fat grafting. A recent survey revealed that 2 mm cannulas (75.8%) with a Mercedes tip (27.3%) were favored by the largest number of providers.[22] The most commonly utilized harvest technique was handheld negative pressure suction aspiration, although powered vacuum suction techniques are also used. In any donor site, harvesting too superficially under the skin or in an uneven distribution can result in unsightly divots or scalloping of the donor region.

The senior author's (JB) preferred technique is to infiltrate the donor site with tumescent solution of 100 cc 0.9% normal saline, 10 cc 0.5% bupivicaine, 20 cc 2% lidocaine, 3 cc 8.4% sodium bicarbonate, 2.4 cc tranexamic acid and 1 cc epinephrine 1:1000. His usual donor sites are the periumbilical lower abdomen, flanks or inner thigh. After the skin is prepared with 4% chlorhexidine sterilization solution, liposuction harvest is effected via a stab incision made with an No.11-blade scalpel, introducing a 2 mm Miller cannula attached to a 10 cc syringe. Handheld negative pressure is applied to the syringe; once collected, the fat is kept upright with the syringe tip pointing down to allow for passive separation of the contents. (See Video 1).

Processing

The optimal technique by which fat is processed has long been debated and currently no gold standard exists. In the past, the most popular method involved centrifugation, although concerns have been raised regarding adipocyte injury which may contribute to variability in fat retention.[24] A recent survey suggested that decantation is being used more readily, a method that avoids force-induced damage to fat cells but unfortunately may have poorer overall efficacy.[22] Some providers purify fat by rolling it in non-adherent cotton pads (Telfa; Covidien, Dublin, Ireland) with or without additional emulsification steps.

In recent years, filtration-based methods, including REVOLVE (LifeCell Corporation, Bridgewater, NJ) and PureGraft (Bimini HealthTech,

Plano, TX), have become available. Purifying harvested material of white blood cells, serum and lysed adipocytes is thought to minimize bruising and post-procedural inflammation, while promoting graft uptake.[24]

Finally, sizing the adipocytes has also been shown to improve uptake and consistency of cosmesis with grafting. Devices such as PureGraft Boost (Bimini HealthTech, Plano, TX) Micronizer and Adinizer (Samson Medical Technologies, Australia) are capable of sizing fat to 1500, 1200, 1000 or 500 micron sizes, depending on the selected filter (See Video 1). Some experts differentiate between fractionated versus unfractionated fat in a manner analogous to high versus low G' injectable hyaluronic acid filler.[25] It has been proposed that larger unfractionated (macro) fat (1.5-2 mm) be injected in a deep preperiosteal plane and smaller fractionated (micro) fat (1 mm) be reserved for more superficial compartments, especially in the periorbital area.

Transfer Technique

After fat is isolated and processed, grafts are transferred into 1 cc syringes. A sharp 18-gauge needle can be used to make a skin opening to introduce the fat injection through the skin (See Video 1). Cannula size selection generally relates to the specific treatment area. Linear feathering or fanning enables retrograde delivery of small volumes of fat into surrounding native tissue, promoting graft survival and a smooth transition between anatomic regions. Transfer details for specific facial regions will be discussed in the subsequent sections. Finally, there exists a dichotomy of opinion relating to timing of fat transfer with concurrent procedures, for instance before or after lower lid blepharoplasty. Some providers maintain that fat should be injected prior to surgical manipulation of the tissue to have enhanced control over its final position. These theories have yet to be substantiated.

TREATMENT REGIONS: UPPER THIRD OF THE FACE

With respect to the upper facial third, forehead height and width are greater in men than in women, with supraorbital bossing and a more abrupt transition to the convex upper forehead.[26] The glabellar prominence is also wider and more projected. The temple is the most frequent location of autologous fat transfer in the upper third, followed by the glabella and then lateral brow. Caution should be exercised when injecting around the brow and periorbital complex due to their proximity to the globe; sharp cannulas should be avoided and surgeons should use their non-dominant hand to protect the globe.

Forehead & Temple

In the temple, fat grafting can provide high levels of patient satisfaction in improvement of hollowing. A recent review of temple rejuvenation described injecting at a variety of tissue depths including superficial to the deep temporal fascia and subcutaneous.[27] A stab incision can be made in the inferolateral temporal hairline just above the zygomatic arch; fat is injected by filling the temporal hollow with fanning toward the hairline. It is important to inject men more cephalically toward the temporal fusion line because they tend to be squarer in the temples rather than round, as seen in females. Some authors advocate for up to 5 to 7 ccs for each temple.[28] The senior author uses an 18-gauge cannula, usually 2 to 3 ccs of fat per side (**Fig. 1**A). Special care must be taken when instrumenting the anterior half of the lower temporal compartment and to avoid major vessels.[27]

Brow, Glabella & Upper Periorbital Complex

Ideal aesthetics of the male brow include a thicker, flatter contour, a gentle peak in the lateral third, and the medial head sitting at or just below the supraorbital rim.[26] The male upper eyelid crease lies lower than females, they have less pretarsal show and their eyes tend to appear more deep set. Whereas a youthful brow and upper eyelid possess fullness

and convexity, aging results in recession of underlying bone, loss of fullness in the glabella and nasion with relatively larger appearance of the nose, dematochalasis, preferential loss of lateral upper eyelid fat and brow ptosis.

Fat grafting to the brow can be performed via a single port at the lateral extent of a blepharoplasty incision in the case of concurrent procedures or via a small stab incision at the inferolateral brow. A blunt cannula should be used to inject 0.5 to 1 cc of fat in a preperiosteal plane at the central and lateral aspects,[28] making the brow more masculine while providing a mild lift (see **Fig. 1**A). Treatment of a hollowed upper eyelid sulcus should be done immediately under the supraorbital rim margin.[28] If a brow lift is done in advance of the fat grafting, it may be difficult to place fat at the desired level, hence special attention to the timing in these cases should be strongly considered.

Grafting the glabella and nasion is done for anti-aging as well as contouring in adjunct to rhinoplasty.[29] In men, this area requires larger volumes, usually between 2-4 cc's (see **Fig. 1**A).[8] This can be done via a medial brow incision or one disguised in a horizontal rhytid of the midline forehead.

TREATMENT REGIONS: MIDDLE THIRD OF THE FACE

In youth, the lower eyelid is shorter with a high lid-cheek transition point. As aging progresses, the

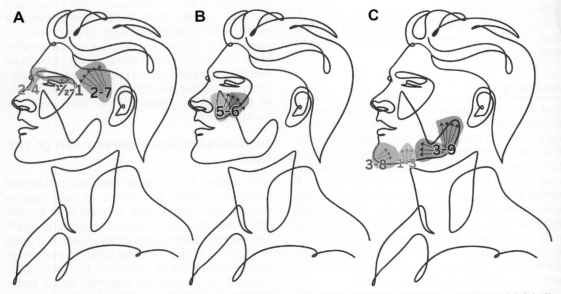

Fig. 1. Average approximate fat augmentation volumes for the male face in the A. Upper facial third (Glabella, *cyan*; Orbital rim/Brow, *green*; Temple, *blue*), (*B*) Middle facial third (Infraorbital complex, *cyan*; Cheek, *Blue*) 3, (*C*) Lower facial third (Chin, *green*; Pre-jowl sulcus, *cyan*; Mandible, *blue*).

lower eyelid becomes longer, with a lower transition point, pseudoherniation of orbital fat and prominent tear troughs. Hypertrophy of the orbicularis oculi pars palpebralis is common.[7] Male volume loss can be more pronounced in the periocular area with them developing more severe lower eyelid skin sagging compared to women.[3] Approach to midfacial injection relies largely on the surgeon's knowledge of the superficial and deep facial fat compartments.[19,20,25] Again, protection of the globe in this region with the surgeon's nondominant hand is highly important.

Tear Troughs & Lower Periorbital Complex

Treatment of the under eye and tear trough should target specific hollowing in nasojugal and/or orbitomalar grooves. The ultimate goal is effacement of the lid-cheek junction, although some persistent definition is more acceptable in male than female patients. The placement of fat in this area should be immediately preperiosteal. Some experts specify the exclusive use of fractionated fat in these areas given the thin and less forgiving overlying skin.[25]

Midface & Cheek

The male cheek tends to contain less volume with a flatter, less rounded appearance.[5] In women, Hinderer's method allows prediction of the zygomaxillary apex; however, in males the malar eminence is more anteromedially positioned and less prominent, while the zygomatic arch is heavier and more inferior.[7] Cheek volumization should reinforce the anterolateral support as excessive volume replacement in the medial compartment tends to age the cheek further. Injections along the zygomatic arch should be lower and with less volume than in women.

Access to the middle third is obtained at the level of the mid-cheek via a stab incision just inferior to the malar eminence and/or just lateral to the alar-facial groove. The senior author routinely grafts patients for whom he performs lower-eyelid blepharoplasty (**Fig. 2**) and indeed many experts advocate for the same.[30–32] He first makes a stab incision using an 18-gauge needle at the level of the malar prominence. Using a 20-gauge cannula, he delivers 2 to 3 cc deeply to the infraorbital complex at the level of the orbital rim and medial malar area in fan-shaped passes (**Fig. 1**B; see Video 1). He then uses a 19-gauge cannula to deep cheek fat pad directly on the bone as well as layering more superficially over the malar prominence and zygoma again 2 to 3 ccs (see **Fig. 1**B; see Video 1)

TREATMENT REGIONS: LOWER THIRD OF THE FACE

The lower third of the face in males is central to their perceived attractiveness.[33] The mandible tends to be larger, more sharply angled and the chin more squared, with prominent square lateral tubercles compared to the gradual taper of the female facial silhouette. Anterior projection of the chin should be centered between two imaginary lines dropped from the oral commissures, while female chin projection should be centered on two imaginary lines dropped from the nasal alar bases. Resorption of the mandible and the descent of the superficial mid-facial fat compartments lead to the loss of jawline definition, jowling and excess submental skin and/or fat.[34] Men tend to prioritize sculpting their chin and jawline, with fewer complaints relating to the perioral area and lips.[33]

Jawline and Chin

To restore a squarer, angular appearance, the cannula is directed superiorly in the direction of the ramus from the mandibular angle. This is in contrast to females, where the cannula is used to sweep along the mandibular angle, directed toward the earlobe.[34] From the same entry point at the angle, the cannula can be directed anteriorly to further define the jawline. Fat is placed in a sub-masseteric/preperiosteal plane, avoiding being subcutaneous, in the parotid or in the masseter.[35] Filling the pre-jowl groove can help create an uninterrupted aesthetic line from chin to the posterior mandible. Here, fat is placed in all tissue layers between the periosteum and skin with approximately 1 to 3 cc on each side (**Fig. 1**C). Millifat or microfat injection may be performed for jawline rejuvenation. Between 3 to 9 cc may be used on each side in total (see **Fig. 1**C).[35]

Fat grafting as a primary method of chin augmentation can be successful for mild microgenia.[21] In a study by Basile and Basile, 42 patients underwent chin augmentation by fat grafting and showed an average increase of 8.9 mm and 7 mm after 4 weeks and 6 months, respectively.[36] The total volume increased averaged 8 cc after 4 weeks and 7.4 cc after 6 months. On average 7.5 cc of fat was injected (see **Fig. 1**C) with an average absorption rate of 17.7%. Grafting to the chin is accessed at the point of desired augmentation, injecting preperiosteally and continuing subcutaneously.[21]

Neck

The aging neck demonstrates skin laxity, horizontal neck lines and lipodystrophy. While there is an increase in subplatysmal fat, there is concurrent loss

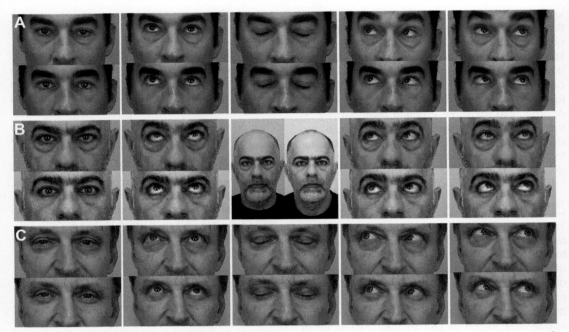

Fig. 2. (*A–C*) Preoperative (*above*) and postoperative (*below*) images of lower blepharoplasty with autologous fat grafting to the cheek, malar and infraorbital follows. Note the universal improvement of the lid-cheek junction without an overdone or operated appearance.

of subdermal fat and dermal aging. Retaining ligaments weaken and allow for descent of the muscle, banding and a more oblique cervicomental angle.[21] In the attractive youthful male neck, the submental-cervical angle should be around 100°, the lateral submandibular-cervical angle around 120 and the posterior submandibular-cervical angle around 140.[37]

Traditionally, neck rejuvenation employed surgical procedures, such as a lower face and neck lift, to recreate the ideal angles. However, non-surgical methods like fat grafting can play an important role, either as an adjunct or standalone procedure. Removing fat in the neck and tightening platysma does not improve the skin quality and when performed in excess, may look unnatural or hollow.[21] Microfat grafting techniques (2 to 4 cc) can be used to fill contour deformities and horizontal neck lines. The microfat should be injected in a subdermal or superficial subcutaneous plane. Nanofat grafting (2 to 6 cc) may be performed to improve skin elasticity and texture. This can be done at 4 to 8 month intervals.[21]

CLINICAL OUTCOMES & COMPLICATIONS

Outcomes assessment from fat grafting typically involves standard comparison of pre- and post-treatment clinical photography. There is no standardized grading for fat grafting treatment outcomes; however, some subjective patient scales have been used to assess persistent hollowness, etc. With the expectation of 30% to 50% reabsorption, final results can be expected by about 6 months as the injected fat cells develop a new blood supply. The primary drawback of autologous fat grafting is the high absorption rate. Thus, fat retention is considered as an essential indicator of procedural success.

Men have a higher risk of bruising post-procedurally possibly due to increased density of facial vasculature,[38,39] a phenomenon that has also been frequently reported in facelift surgery. Acutely, fat grafting can result in hematoma, seroma, infection and nerve injury. In the longer term, issues with textural irregularities, calcifications, and oil cysts can occur and are occasionally reasons for revision.[39] The most dreaded complication of autologous fat grafting is similar to that of injectable filler, that is, intra-arterial injection. A recent systematic review of the literature that was published in Aesthetic Plastic Surgery[40] identified 61 reported events, most commonly involving injections targeting the glabella or multiple facial regions (26.2%) followed by injections in the temples (16.4%) and lastly the forehead (14.8%). There is currently no evidence to suggest that male patients would be at higher risk for this particular complication.

SUMMARY

Fat grafting of the male face is an excellent tool for facial rejuvenation either as an adjunct or a stand-alone procedure. Sensitivity regarding the nature of aging changes unique to the male face as well as understanding men's unique aesthetic goals will allow the skilled practitioner to tailor rejuvenating treatments accordingly.

CLINICS CARE POINTS

- The facial plastic surgeon must have a firm understanding of skeletal and soft-tissue anatomic divergences, as well as unique biologic and histologic features, relating to each gender
- Fat grafting can be used for structural enhancement of male facial features that may wane with aging, namely the mandible, chin, brow and midface. It can improve skin quality in areas like the neck.
- Targeted augmentation with fat should be performed carefully to avoid feminizing the face
- Males are at increased risk for bruising and bleeding from facial cosmetic procedures, including fat grafting

DISCLOSURE

Dr J.D. Bloom is a consultant and speaker's bureau member for Bimini HealthTech & Suneva. Dr E.C. Deane and Dr A. Wong have no financial interest to declare in relation to the context of this article.

SUPPLEMENTARY DATA

Supplementary data related to this article can be found online at https://doi.org/10.1016/j.fsc.2024.03.003.

REFERENCES

1. Aesthetic Plastic Surgery National Databank Statistics 2020-2021. Aesthet Surg J 2022;42(Suppl 1):1–18.
2. Fabi S, Alexiades M, Chatrath V, et al. Facial Aesthetic Priorities and Concerns: A Physician and Patient Perception Global Survey. Aesthet Surg J 2022;42(4):NP218–29.
3. Cohen BE, Bashey S, Wysong A. Literature Review of Cosmetic Procedures in Men: Approaches and Techniques are Gender Specific. Am J Clin Dermatol 2017;18(1):87–96.
4. Sadick NS. Volumetric Structural Rejuvenation for the Male Face. Dermatol Clin 2018;36(1):43–8.
5. Bass LS. Cheek Shaping with Implants and Fillers. In: Steinbrech D, editor. Male Aesthetic Plastic Surgery. New York: Thieme Publishers; 2020. p. 187–99. https://doi.org/10.1055/b-0040-178155.
6. Dhaliwal J, Friedman O. Injectables and Fillers in Male Patients. Facial Plast Surg Clin N Am 2008; 16(3):345–55.
7. de Maio M. Ethnic and Gender Considerations in the Use of Facial Injectables: Male Patients. Plast Reconstr Surg 2015;136(5 Suppl):40S–3S.
8. Coleman SR. Chapter 14 Facial Fat Grafting in Men. In: Steinbrech D, editor. Male Aesthetic Plastic Surgery. New York: Thieme Publishers; 2020. p. 143–85. https://doi.org/10.1055/b-0040-178155.
9. Clauser LC, Tieghi R, Galiè M, et al. Structural fat grafting: facial volumetric restoration in complex reconstructive surgery. J Craniofac Surg 2011; 22(5):1695–701.
10. Giacomoni PU, Mammone T, Teri M. Gender-linked differences in human skin. J Dermatol Sci 2009; 55(3):144–9.
11. Somenek M. Gender-Related Facial Surgical Goals. Facial Plast Surg FPS 2018;34(5):474–9.
12. Wan D, Amirlak B, Giessler P, et al. The differing adipocyte morphologies of deep versus superficial midfacial fat compartments: a cadaveric study. Plast Reconstr Surg 2014;133(5):615e–22e.
13. Lakhiani C, Somenek MT. Gender-related Facial Analysis. Facial Plast Surg Clin N Am 2019;27(2): 171–7.
14. Farhadian JA, Bloom BS, Brauer JA. Male Aesthetics: A Review of Facial Anatomy and Pertinent Clinical Implications. J Drugs Dermatol JDD 2015; 14(9):1029–34.
15. Mendelson B, Wong CH. Changes in the facial skeleton with aging: implications and clinical applications in facial rejuvenation. Aesthetic Plast Surg 2012;36(4):753–60.
16. Leong PL. Aging changes in the male face. Facial Plast Surg Clin N Am 2008;16(3):277–9.
17. Tsukahara K, Hotta M, Osanai O, et al. Gender-dependent differences in degree of facial wrinkles. Skin Res Technol 2013;19(1):e65–71.
18. Rohrich RJ, Avashia YJ, Savetsky IL. Prediction of Facial Aging Using the Facial Fat Compartments. Plast Reconstr Surg 2021;147(1S-2):38S–42S.
19. Ramanadham SR, Rohrich RJ. Newer Understanding of Specific Anatomic Targets in the Aging Face as Applied to Injectables: Superficial and Deep Facial Fat Compartments–An Evolving Target for Site-Specific Facial Augmentation. Plast Reconstr Surg 2015;136(5 Suppl):49S–55S.
20. Wan D, Amirlak B, Rohrich R, et al. The clinical importance of the fat compartments in midfacial aging. Plast Reconstr Surg Glob Open 2013;1(9):e92.

21. Azoury SC, Shakir S, Bucky LP, et al. Modern Fat Grafting Techniques to the Face and Neck 2021; 148(4).

22. Vizcay M, Saha S, Mohammad A, et al. Current Fat Grafting Practices and Preferences: A Survey from Members of ISPRES. Plast Reconstr Surg Glob Open 2023;11(3):e4849.

23. Ismail T, Bürgin J, Todorov A, et al. Low osmolality and shear stress during liposuction impair cell viability in autologous fat grafting. J Plast Reconstr Aesthetic Surg JPRAS 2017;70(5):596–605.

24. Fang C, Patel P, Li H, et al. Physical, Biochemical, and Biologic Properties of Fat Graft Processed via Different Methods. Plast Reconstr Surg Glob Open 2020;8(8):e3010.

25. Rodriguez-Unda NA, Novak MD, Rohrich RJ. Techniques in Facial Fat Grafting: Optimal Results Based on the Science of Facial Aging. Plast Reconstr Surg 2023e010314.   https://doi.org/10.1097/PRS. 0000000000010314.

26. Sedgh J. The Aesthetics of the Upper Face and Brow: Male and Female Differences. Facial Plast Surg FPS 2018;34(2):114–8.

27. Othman S, Cohn JE, Burdett J, et al. Temporal Augmentation: A Systematic Review. Facial Plast Surg FPS 2020;36(3):217–25.

28. Tzikas TL. Fat Grafting Volume Restoration to the Brow and Temporal Regions. Facial Plast Surg FPS 2018;34(2):164–72.

29. Kornstein AN, Nikfarjam JS. Fat Grafting to the Forehead/Glabella/Radix Complex and Pyriform Aperture: Aesthetic and Anti-Aging Implications. Plast Reconstr Surg Glob Open 2015;3(8):e500.

30. Rohrich RJ, Ghavami A, Mojallal A. The five-step lower blepharoplasty: blending the eyelid-cheek junction. Plast Reconstr Surg 2011;128(3):775–83.

31. Scheuer JF 3rd, Matarasso A, Rohrich RJ. Optimizing Male Periorbital Rejuvenation. Dermatol Surg Off Publ Am Soc Dermatol Surg Al 2017; 43(Suppl 2):S196–202.

32. Massry GG, Azizzadeh B. Periorbital fat grafting. Facial Plast Surg FPS 2013;29(1):46–57.

33. Mastroluca E, Patalano M, Bertossi D. Minimally invasive aesthetic treatment of male patients: The importance of consultation and the lower third of the face. J Cosmet Dermatol 2021;20(7):2086–92.

34. Vazirnia A, Braz A, Fabi SG. Nonsurgical jawline rejuvenation using injectable fillers. J Cosmet Dermatol 2020;19(8):1940–7.

35. Marten T, Elyassnia D. Facial Fat Grafting: Why, Where, How, and How Much. Aesthetic Plast Surg 2018;42(5):1278–97.

36. Basile FV, Basile AR. Prospective Controlled Study of Chin Augmentation by Means of Fat Grafting. Plast Reconstr Surg 2017;140. https://doi.org/10. 1097/PRS.0000000000003895.

37. Bravo FG. Neck Contouring and Rejuvenation in Male Patients Through Dual-Plane Reduction Neck Lift. Clin Plast Surg 2022;49(2):257–73.

38. Mayrovitz HN, Regan MB. Gender differences in facial skin blood perfusion during basal and heated conditions determined by laser Doppler flowmetry. Microvasc Res 1993;45(2):211–8.

39. Yoshimura K, Coleman SR. Complications of Fat Grafting: How They Occur and How to Find, Avoid, and Treat Them. Clin Plast Surg 2015;42(3):383–8, ix.

40. Moellhoff N, Kuhlmann C, Frank K, et al. Arterial Embolism After Facial Fat Grafting: A Systematic Literature Review. Aesthetic Plast Surg 2023. https://doi. org/10.1007/s00266-023-03511-y.

Contemporary Male Rhinoplasty Surgery

Ivan Wayne, MD[a,b,*]

KEYWORDS

- Male rhinoplasty • Rhinoplasty • Preservation rhinoplasty • Male aesthetic surgery
- Functional rhinoplasty

KEY POINTS

- The goals of male rhinoplasty patients may differ from those of females. Male patients typically desire more conservative results.
- The motivations of male patients seeking rhinoplasty surgery needs a more in-depth evaluation than that of the typically female patient, as there are potential psycho-social issues that will impact expectations and patient satisfaction.
- The male patient may have greater difficult adapting to changes in appearance during the healing phase after surgery and pre-surgical counseling is recommended.
- The nasal tissues of the male patient differ from the female patient, and surgical strategies need to take these differences into account when planning and performing rhinoplasty surgery in this population.
- Male patients seeking rhinoplasty surgery often have more functional concerns and issues than female patients that will need to be treated in combination with any aesthetic improvements.

INTRODUCTION

Rhinoplasty in the male patient presents the surgeon with several unique challenges in addition to all the expected issues one encounters in female rhinoplasty. The experienced rhinoplasty surgeon will often find themselves tensing up when entering the consult room for a prospective male rhinoplasty, having been conditioned by multiple difficult past experiences with this population. In this article we will review some of the issues that may be encountered in this patient population.

Even though exact rhinoplasty numbers by sex have not recently been compiled, the majority (64.7%) are female, placing male rhinoplasty in the minority. In one senior surgeon's reporting the ratio was 23% male and 77% female.[1]

While for the typical surgeon a male rhinoplasty case will be in the minority, these cases bring additional challenges that must be addressed to successfully provide care for these patients.

With the male patient, psychosocial issues are perhaps the most important distinction from female patients, as the pitfalls these present the surgeon are significant and potentially problematic. In the most extreme examples, the safety of the surgeon and their staff are potentially at risk. There have been several instances globally of mentally disturbed male rhinoplasty patients murdering their physicians after a failed surgery. For the surgeon, connecting with and understanding their patients is critically important, as repercussions for failing to do so could have dire consequences. Patient expectations for changes to be achieved can be somewhat nebulous. While the female patient often has clear expectations and will feel comfortable sharing her thoughts and desires during the consultation, the male patient may not be as up front. The male patient may focus on breathing

a Department of Otorhinolaryngology, University of Oklahoma College of Medicine, Oklahoma City, OK, USA;
b W Aesthetics, 10001 Broadway Extension, Suite A, Oklahoma City, OK 73114, USA
* W Aesthetics, 10001 Broadway Extension, Suite A, Oklahoma City, OK 73114.
E-mail address: Ivanwayne@icloud.com

Facial Plast Surg Clin N Am 32 (2024) 399–408
https://doi.org/10.1016/j.fsc.2024.03.004
1064-7406/24/© 2024 Elsevier Inc. All rights reserved.

difficulties or perceived deviation while his actual concern may be strictly aesthetic.[2]

An important fact that the surgeon must keep in mind that men seeking cosmetic surgery have a higher rate of dissatisfaction with their appearance prior to surgery than female patients.[3] As well, male cosmetic surgery patients also have a lower satisfaction rate with their surgery than female patients (56% vs 87.6%)[4]

The male patient can be both demanding and less able to communicate his goals to the surgeon, necessitating a more careful evaluation during the consultation process.[1] Some patient characteristics that can suggest underlying psychiatric issues are listed in **Box 1**[2]

Often, the red flags listed in **Box 1** will present as the patient interacts with the office staff before the actual patient encounter, and the surgeon should investigate these potential issues with staff members who have interacted with them.

Patient age is a significant factor. In the teenager with all the stress factors of social media, body self-awareness and with possible depression and anxiety a significant positive change is often seen after rhinoplasty surgery.[5,6] Typically, the more aged male who often presents with nasal-tip ptosis, thicker sebaceous skin and nasal-valve compromise, a desire for both functional and aesthetic improvements is seen.[7]

Preoperative Consultation

As outlined above, many potential psycho-social issues may be present in men requesting rhinoplasty surgery, and significant time and focus on understanding the patient and his desires/goals during the consultation process is prudent. A good candidate will have reasonable concerns, a noticeable deformity, an ability to communicate and be a well-adjusted individual with a healthy social network. The opposite patient is the male with the "SIMON" complex.[8] The "SIMON" complex is a group of characteristics that stands for Single, Immature, Male, Overly expectant and Narcissistic. While having these traits does not mean the patient is a poor candidate for surgery, they are red flags that should prompt the surgeon to dive more deeply into motivations and expectations during the consultation process. Body dysmorphic syndrome is a more serious red flag for the surgeon, and these patients will not benefit from aesthetic surgery. It behooves the physician to assist these patients in getting the professional support and care they need.[1]

Anatomic analysis includes all the standard features that are addressed in female patients, such as skin thickness, nasal bone projection and width, nasal tip support and position, as well nasolabial angle and internal characteristics. The male patient typically has thicker more sebaceous skin influencing skin re-draping and possible contracture or lack of long-term contracture. When discussing goals with the male patient, it is generally accepted that a straight dorsum with minimal to no nasal tip break is desired, but this must be carefully reviewed with the patient during the consultation process.[1]

As well as dorsal changes, tip rotation needs special attention. In the female patient the optimal nasolabial angle is 95 to 105°, while in the male patient 90° is generally preferred, though once again a clear discussion of expectations and goals needs to be discussed with the patient.[9] The use of imaging software to simulate possible surgical options for proposed dorsal changes and tip rotation can be very useful in clarifying goals with the prospective male rhinoplasty patient.[10]

While occasionally a well-adjusted male seeking rhinoplasty may want something more aggressive than a straight dorsum and refined tip with a minimal break with a 90-degree nasolabial angle, it is generally assumed that this is the aesthetic standard and goal for the male nose.

Box 1
Patient characteristics that can suggest underlying psychiatric issues

Minor disfigurement that the patient is very preoccupied with

A delusion concerning the appearance of the nose

History of multiple rhinoplasty or aesthetic surgeries

Unclear reasons for wanting surgery

Identity conflict

Expectations that surgery could alter other realms of life

History of limited social interaction or difficulty in social and emotional relationships

Currently in a grieving state or crisis situation

Very neurotic and concerned about aging and appearance

Hostile attitude toward staff or the surgeon

History of seeing numerous physicians regarding the patient's primary complaint

Exhibiting paranoia

Low self-esteem

Manipulative, especially with surgeon and staff

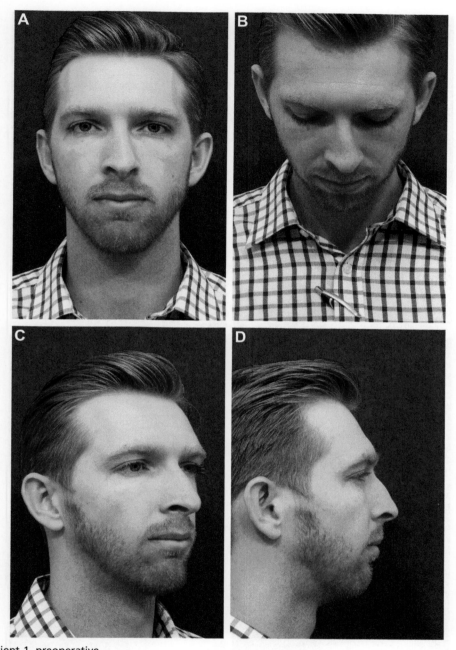

Fig. 1. Patient 1, preoperative.

Anatomic Considerations

The typical male face is heavy and has a squarer shape, with a larger nose overall than in the female face. The male nasal dorsum is wider and straighter as well. The nasal tip is broader and more bulbous. The thicker nasal skin limits the external changes visible after underlying skeletal changes.[11]

Surgical Considerations

Generally, rhinoplasty surgery in the male patient is similar to that in the female patient with a focus on the unique aesthetic goals that have been outlined above. There are several options available with respect to approaches-external versus endonasal (delivery or intra cartilaginous). The choice will depend on the surgeon's comfort

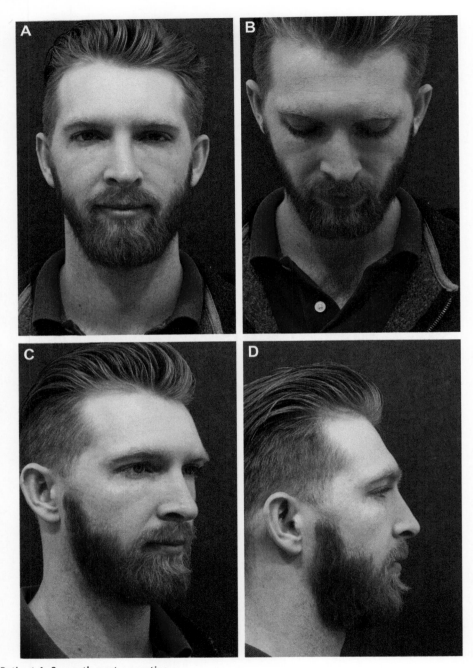

Fig. 2. Patient 1, 9 month post operative.

level and experience as well as the specifics of the case.

With respect to addressing the dorsal hump, typical hump resections, or humpectomies, with rasps or osteotomes are effective and often indicated. The surgeon may choose from several powered instruments (rasps or drills) to both reduce the dorsal height as well thinning the thick nasal bones (rhino-sculpture). The piezo electric device, which can function as both a saw and a rasp may be used, and some surgeons find this a precise and effective instrument for cutting and shaping the nasal bones.[12,13]

More recently, the option to use dorsal preservation to reduce a nasal hump has become popular in Europe and South America, and

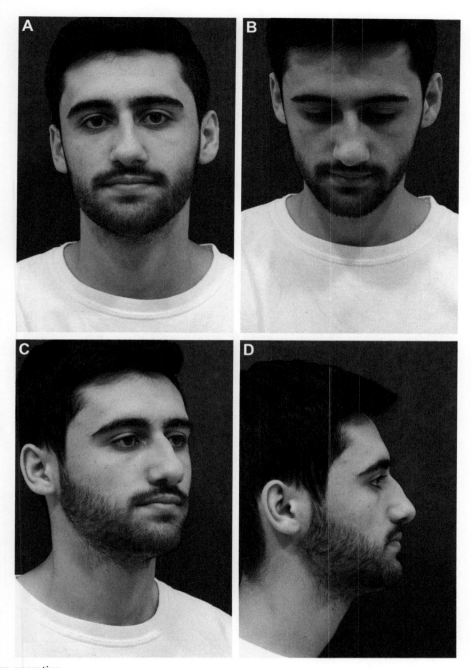

Fig. 3. Pre-operative.

excellent results can be achieved with this technique.

In the author's experience, the male dorsal hump has larger, thicker bones than in the female, and more effort is required to achieve appropriate reduction using the various maneuvers including hump reduction and osteotomy creation. The thicker bones and periosteum in the male patient can be more resistant to cutting during the performance of the lateral osteotomy. Special focus on the lateral osteotomies is prudent as re-lateralization may occur if the bones have not been adequately released and medialized.

After dorsal hump reduction (humpectomy), the middle vault can be reconstructed with spreader grafts or spreader flaps, both of which have been

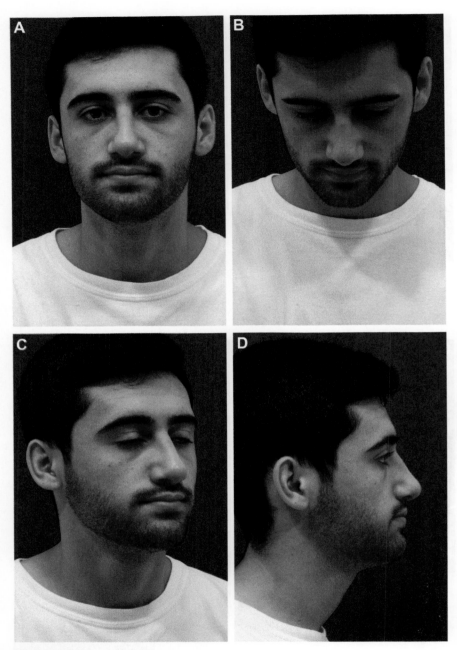

Fig. 4. 6-month post-operative results.

shown to be effective in restoring the middle vault while preserving ideal brow-tip aesthetic lines and hopefully avoiding disruption of the internal valve.[14,15] Alternatively, hump reduction in preservation rhinoplasty completely avoids disruption of the keystone, thereby preserving the integrity of the nasal valve and brow-tip aesthetic lines.[16]

A greater problem in male rhinoplasty that is less common than in the female nose is affecting stable, long-term changes in the nasal tip, both with rotation/projection and tip refinement. This is a result of thicker, less elastic nasal skin. The thicker skin masks changes in the nasal tip cartilages used to refine the width and definition of the nasal tip, and the less elastic skin puts more stress on tip-support mechanisms over time. The recurrent pressure from facial expressions can transmit to the nasal skin and tend to reduce

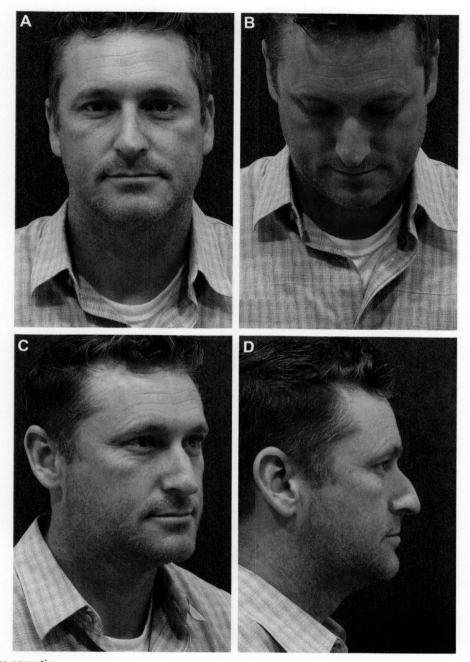

Fig. 5. Pre-operative.

projection and de-rotate the nasal tip over time, so extra attention to re-enforcing nasal tip support and strength is prudent during surgery.

Deviations or weakness in the caudal septum should be addressed prior to setting tip position. Effective maneuvers include the tongue-and-groove technique, columellar strut grafts and septal extension grafts. For long-term stability in the ptotic male tip, the authors have found the use of side-to-side septal extension grafts to be the most reliable method of maintaining stable tip position, locking the graft into the bony nasal spine and securing to the caudal septum for maximal stability. The ideal material for these grafts is autologous septal cartilage. If inadequate septal material is available for grafting, other sources include

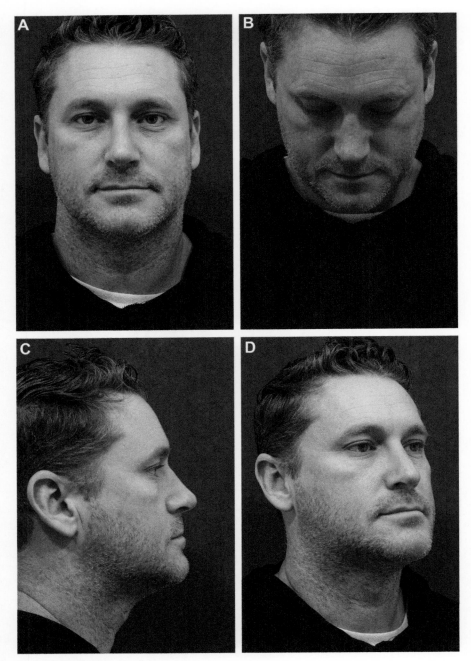

Fig. 6. 7-month post-operative result.

auricular and costal cartilage sites, each with specific pros and cons. Generally, auricular cartilage is quite weak and has significant curvature, making it a poor choice to provide straight, strong nasal tip support over time. Costal cartilage is significantly stronger but has greater donor-site challenges and working with these grafts is more involved. There is also the possibility of calcification of the rib, making both harvest and shaping more difficult, though the new piezo electric cutting instruments can help with this task. Some surgeons routinely use irradiated cadaver donor costal rib cartilage and have reported good long-term results using this option.[17,18]

The nasal tip in the male patient is subject to greater stresses than the female nose with the thicker nasal skin weighing it down. There is also a significant flattening force on the nasal tip during the action of smiling. These deforming forces from the facial mimetic muscles in the less elastic male face are greater than in the typical female face. These increased stresses necessitate the need for strong support, and moderate over correction of tip position "on the table" is often indicated. The need to create strong tip support and possible over correction should be discussed with the patient during the pre-operative planning phase and counseling as to the expected changes that are likely to occur as the swelling resolves and the nasal tip settles in. The typical male who may be unaccustomed to radical changes in his appearance may be shocked at how dramatically his nose changes after a rhinoplasty prior to final healing that can take months.

Post-operative care is routine in the male patient. Swelling will often be pronounced with thicker nasal skin, and the edema may be more persistent. Prolonged edema in the skin soft-tissue envelope may lead to secondary deformities, most often in the supra-tip area where thickening and fibrosis can occur in the thick-skinned male patient. The surgeon may consider taping therapy or triamcinolone injections in recalcitrant cases.[19,20] Patient 1 is a 28-year-old male with a dorsal hump, deviated dorsum and septum with significant nasal obstruction (**Fig. 1**A-D).

Case 1: Patient 1 is a 28-year-old male with a dorsal hump, deviated dorsum and septum with significant nasal obstruction. He desires reduction of the dorsal hump and straightening of the bridge as well correction of the functional issues. He underwent an open septo-rhinoplasty with component hump reduction, lateral and paramedium osteotomies (en-bloc) to correct the deviated bony dorsum. Asymmetric spreader flaps (right > left) were used to reconstruct the middle vault and a unilateral side-to-side septal extension graft harvested from the septum was used to support the tip in a tongue-and-groove fashion with medial crural footpads.

This case illustrates the challenges of rhinoplasty in the severely crooked nose. Achieving a straight nose when both the nose and nasal base/pyriform aperture are deviated is often not possible. Patient was counseled pre-operatively and pleased with his result (**Fig. 2**).

Case 2: Patient 2 is a 22-year-old male with a dorsal hump, deviated dorsum and a wide bulbous nasal tip desiring improvement in nasal deviation and reduction of the dorsal hump. This nose was treated with a dorsal hump reduction, right-sided spreader graft, unilateral side-to-side septal extension graft, and the tip position was secured with the tongue-and-groove technique. Tip reduction achieved with dome suturing and articulating alar-rim grafts. Dorsal deviation addressed with en-bloc osteotomy and unilateral right-sided spreader graft (**Figs. 3–5**).

Case 3: 47-year-old patient presents with nasal obstruction secondary to a deviated septum and nasal valve compromise. He has a significant dorsal hump and pronounced dorsal deviation. He has severe tip ptosis and under projection. Patient desires improvement in breathing and conservative aesthetic refinement and a straighter nose.

A septo-rhinoplasty was performed with a dorsal hump reduction, asymmetric spreader flaps, L > R, a unilateral side-to-side septal extension graft secured to the medial crural footpads in the tongue-and-groove fashion, projecting and rotating the nasal tip. Dorsal deviation addressed with the en-bloc osteotomy and asymmetric spreader flaps (**Fig. 6**).

SUMMARY

With careful patient selection after consideration and attention to the unique psycho-social issues and challenges of the male rhinoplasty patient combined with appropriate counseling, these patients can achieve successful outcomes with improved nasal function and aesthetics.

DISCLOSURE

Authors have nothing to disclose.

REFERENCES

1. Simons RL, Adelson RT. Rhinoplasty in male patients. Facial Plast Surg 2005;21:240–9.
2. Rohrich RJ, Mohan R. Male Rhinoplasty: Update. Plast Reconstr Surg 2020;145(4):744e–53e.
3. Winkler AA, Downs BW. Aging male rhinoplasty. Facial Plast Surg Clin North Am 2008;16:329–35, vi.
4. Khansa I, Khansa L, Pearson GD. Patient satisfaction after rhinoplasty: A social media analysis. Aesthet Surg J 2016;36:NP1–5.
5. McGrath MH, Mukerji S. Plastic surgery and the teenage patient. J Pediatr Adolesc Gynecol 2000; 13:105–18.
6. Chauhan N, Warner J, Adamson PA. Adolescent rhinoplasty: challenges and psychosocial and clinical outcomes. Aesthetic Plast Surg 2010;34:510–6.
7. Cochran CS, Ducic Y, DeFatta RJ. Restorative rhinoplasty in the aging patient. Laryngoscope 2007;117: 803–7.
8. Gorney M. Cosmetic surgery in males. Plast Reconstr Surg 2002;110:719.
9. Sinno HH, Markarian MK, Ibrahim AM, et al. The ideal nasolabial angle in rhinoplasty: a preference

analysis of the general population. Plast Reconstr Surg 2014;134:201–10.

10. Mühlbauer W, Holm C. Computer Imaging and Surgical Reality in Aesthetic Rhinoplasty. Plast Reconstr Surg 2005;115(7):2098–104.

11. Rohrich RJ, Janis JE, Gunter JP, et al. Male rhinoplasty. In: Dallas rhinoplasty: nasal surgery by the Masters. 2nd edition. St Louis: Quality Medical Publishing; 2007. p. 1281–304.

12. Gerbault O, Daniel RK, Kosins AM. The role of piezo-electric instrumentation in rhinoplasty surgery. Aesthet Surg J 2016;36(1):21–34.

13. Racy E, Fanous A, Benmoussa N. Powered Rhinoplasty: A Simple Step-by-Step Approach. Plast Reconstr Surg 2021;147(1):65–7.

14. Sheen JH. Spreader graft: A method of reconstructing the roof of the middle nasal vault following rhinoplasty. Plast Reconstr Surg 1984;73:230–9.

15. Rohrich RJ, Durand P. Four-Step Spreader Flap: The Pull-Twist-Turn Technique. Plastic and Reconstructive Surg 2021;147(3):608–12.

16. Toriumi DM, Kovacevic M, Kosins AM. Structural Preservation Rhinoplasty: A Hybrid Approach. Plast Reconstr Surg 2022;149(5):1105–20.

17. Rohrich RJ, Abraham J, Alleyne B, et al. Fresh Frozen Rib Cartilage Grafts in Revision Rhinoplasty: A 9-Year Experience. Plast Reconstr Surg 2022;150(1):58–62.

18. Kridel RW, Ashoori F, Liu ES, et al. Long-term use and follow-up of irradiated homologous costal cartilage grafts in the nose. Archives Facial Plast Surg 2009;11(6):378–94.

19. Anderson JR. Symposium. Laryngoscope 1976;86(1):53–7.

20. Guyuron B, DeLuca L, Lash R. Supratip Deformity: A Closer Look. Plast Reconstr Surg 2000;105(3):1140–51.

Facial Hair in Hair Restoration Surgery
Beard Transplantation and Beard-To-Scalp Hair Restoration

Jeffrey S. Epstein, MD

KEYWORDS

- Beard transplant • Facial hair restoration • FUE hair restoration • Mustache transplant • BHT

KEY POINTS

- Beard restoration requires meticulous acute angulation of grafts and aesthetic design. In a typical procedure, 2200 to 2800 grafts are typically indicated.
- In most beard restoration cases, grafts containing one and two hairs are used, so naturally occurring three or more hair grafts require division.
- Meticulous graft dissection to remove the surrounding skin cuff significantly reduces the risk of bump formation around each graft, of particular importance to grafts placed in the chin mound and soul-patch region.
- Beard hairs can effectively be transplanted into the scalp, a procedure called body hair transplantation. This is indicated in cases of advanced hair loss or in reparative cases that present with a limited donor supply of scalp hairs for transplantation.
- Follicular unit excision removal procedures are the most effective approach to repair the poor aesthetic results from poorly executed prior beard transplantation.

INTRODUCTION

Twenty-one years ago in these Facial Plastic Surgery Clinics, in the early days of these specialized procedures, I coauthored an article on nonscalp hair restoration.[1] In subsequent years the popularity of beard restoration soared. In the mid-2000s the popular Brooklyn "hipster" trend included a beard as a defining characteristic, a trend that is now embraced by society. Another demographic trend is the growing popularity of gender reaffirmation, with some female-to-male patients now seeking fuller beards than that which can be achieved by exogenous hormones alone. An important technical development that has fed the procedure growth is the refinement of the follicular unit excision (FUE) technique. FUE procedures make possible the combination of a full beard and shaved head without the donor-site scar resulting from the follicular unit transplantation (FUT or "strip") technique.

With an increasing number of physicians performing beard and scalp restoration procedures, and in increasing number of procedures being performed, an associated increase in the need for corrective procedures occurs. This increase led to two other developments: the use of FUE removal to repair beard transplant and body hair transplantation (BHT) where beard hairs serve as donor hairs for scalp restoration in cases of insufficient scalp-hair donor supply.

Patient Candidacy and Indications

Beard restoration is performed on men seeking more facial hair. In most cases, the patient never had the desired amount of facial hair, but

Department of Otolaryngology, University of Miami, 6280 Sunset Drive, Suite 504, Miami, FL 33143, USA
E-mail address: jse@drjeffreyepstein.com

Facial Plast Surg Clin N Am 32 (2024) 409–416
https://doi.org/10.1016/j.fsc.2024.02.005
1064-7406/24/© 2024 Elsevier Inc. All rights reserved.

occasionally the condition is due to prior laser hair removal. Other causes include scarring alopecia such as from cleft palate, lesion-removal surgery, or radiation therapy. Further, beard senescence and the graying of beard hair may cause the beard to lose some of its appearance of density. This issue can be improved by transplanting darker scalp hairs. In all of these cases, procedures ranging from several hundred to as many as 2500 or more grafts can be transplanted in a single-day procedure.

Scalp hairs are the most common donors for beard restoration because of their high reliability in regrowth, natural look once transplanted, and availability in large quantities. Patients must be counseled that if they desire scalp hair restoration in the future their scalp hair donor availability will be affected by their beard transplantation. In certain cases beard hairs can be used as donor hair, particularly in smaller cases (several hundred or fewer grafts) such as those performed to reinforce the mustache or fill patchiness in the cheek beard. Most commonly, the desired hairs are harvested from below the jawline where these missing hairs will go unnoticed.

A different but related procedure is BHT in which beard hairs are used for restoring scalp hair. BHT is a relatively new tool in the armamentarium of hair restoration surgeons, made possible by the more advanced FUE drill systems that overcome many of the challenges in beard hair harvesting. These challenges include ergonomics, skin quality, and hair fragility.[2,3] Beard donor hairs, once placed into the scalp, have a high regrowth rate, and these typically coarser and thicker hairs retain their thickness but largely lose their coarseness. This phenomenon permits their use even in the more visible zones of the scalp including toward the hairline. Beard donor-site punch holes heal rapidly, typically taking only 24 hours as compared with the 3 days for scalp donor areas. In most cases, it is possible to harvest 800 to 1200 grafts from under the jawline in a single procedure without causing any noticeable decrease in density.

Patient candidacy for beard restoration is not limited by age, skin complexion, nor ethnicity. **Figs. 1–3** show the results of beard restoration in a Caucasian, Asian, and Black patient. Although there are tremendous variations in skin color, hair texture and curl, and skin healing, these three examples demonstrate the possibility for achieving naturalness in a multitude of patients.[4,5] The typical Asian patient presents challenges in beard restoration due to the tendency of rigidly straight scalp donor hairs thick in caliber. Further, there is significant contrast between light skin color and dark hairs. Successful results occur with meticulous graft placement and angulation combined with the use of mostly, if not all, single and occasional two-hair grafts. Asian patients are frequently counseled that they may desire a second procedure to achieve sufficient density. In Black patients, curly hairs require larger recipient sites (0.6 mm vs the more typical 0.5 mm) for one- and two-hair grafts. Dense graft packing is more challenging, but fortunately these curly hairs are frequently amenable to some three-hair graft placement, with results both natural-appearing and maximally dense. Prior concerns of folliculitis and hyperpigmentation in these cases have not proved true.

The female-to-male gender reaffirmation patient can attain a much fuller beard with hair transplantation than that typically achieved with hormonal supplementation alone.[6] These patients, much like any younger male, need to be advised of their risk of future male pattern hair loss, with the reduction in scalp-hair donor supply for future transplantation into areas of scalp hair loss. Meanwhile, the male-to-female gender reaffirmation patient is one of the best possible candidates for BHT beard-to-scalp hair harvesting due to the presence of what are now undesirable beard hairs. If counseled early, instead of laser hair removal, the male-to-female patient with advanced male pattern hair loss can have thousands of beard hairs harvested to contribute to scalp coverage.

Cleft lip and other scars in the beard region are appropriately concealed with hair transplantation. Patients are advised, similar to scalp scars, of the risk of a lower percentage of hair regrowth. To overcome this risk, several steps can be taken to enhance hair regrowth in the scar, including deeper recipient sites, transplanting into mature scar (at least 12–18 months), using mostly two- and even three-hair grafts, and injecting platelet rich plasma at the time of the procedure. **Fig. 4** shows an example of facial scarring treated with hair grafting.

There are several facial hair zones: the sideburns, the cheek beards, the mustache, the goatee (that in some classifications includes the mustache), and that portion below the jawline. The cheek beards and sideburns are the two zones easiest in which to attain natural and impressive results with transplants.[7] To achieve moderate density in cases of minimal existing original hairs, each sideburn requires 200 to 250 grafts per side and each cheek beard, 350 to 550 grafts per side depending on the height of the beard line. The mustache is clearly the most challenging area. The pink lip protrusion line and the philtrum indentation, or "cupid's bow", increase the difficulty of site placement.[4]

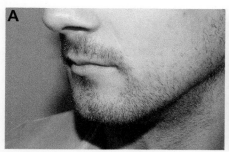 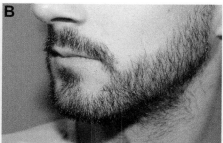

Fig. 1. Before (*A*) and 1 year after (*B*) a beard transplant procedure of 1900 grafts in a Caucasian patient.

Achieving moderate density in the mustache requires 300 to 400 grafts. Finally, the completion of the goatee includes the chin mound and requires 300 to 400 grafts, whereas the "soul patch" or the small patch of hair directly under the lower lip requires 50 to 150 grafts. These two areas are difficult areas in which to achieve thick density and also at greatest risk for developing bumps around each graft when the skin surrounding the hairs has been insufficiently trimmed. Extension below the jawline can be performed in those patients who desire this coverage, but this may not be the most effective use of what are often limited quantities of donor hairs.

Consultation with the patient can be done either in person or virtually, as well as by photographic review. It is possible for patients to return to public as soon as 1 or 2 days later wearing a mask, and by 5 to 6 days, most patients are fully presentable. Shaving of the beard in the recipient-site area is permitted 10 days postprocedure, whereas the donor area of the beard may be shaved 1 week postprocedure. Younger patients, at risk of developing male pattern hair loss, must be advised that any grafts used in the beard will be unavailable for transplantation into the scalp, thereby reducing the amount of possible coverage. With the advancement in FUE techniques, patients can have both a shaved head and a full beard, a commonly desired look. If patients desire

additional density with a second procedure, this can be performed as early as 8 months later. Patients with light skin and dark, fine hair may be particularly interested in this option.

The Surgery

Primary beard transplantation

Design and graft counts Design is typically guided by the patient, who demonstrates his goals with online photos. Multiple options are possible, including a limited amount of goatee coverage, a narrow strap beard, a thick mustache, a full thick "lumberjack"-appearing beard with high borders, and extension in the goatee up to the lower lip line.

Required graft counts are determined by the following: the areas to be filled; the desired density; the preexisting number of beard hairs; and the donor-hair characteristics that include color, thickness/caliber, curl, and average hairs per follicular unit. Some general rules of anticipated graft counts are displayed in **Table 1**.

It is possible to transplant 4000 grafts into the beard in a single procedure taking one and a half days. On day one the goatee and central cheek regions are transplanted with 2700 to 3000 grafts, typically the maximum that can be transplanted into the facial region in a single day. The balance are then transplanted on the second day. However, a more conservative approach is generally recommended. A typical male has 6500 to 7000 total

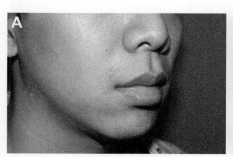 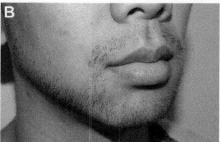

Fig. 2. Before (*A*) and 1 year after (*B*) a beard transplant procedure of 1800 grafts in a Black patient.

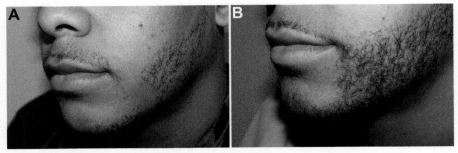

Fig. 3. Before (*A*) and 1 year after (*B*) a beard transplant procedure of 1400 grafts in an Asian patient. In this case, the patient desired a subtle creation of a "strap" beard.

FUE grafts to donate before the donor area appears patchy. Note, however, that because in most cases of beard hair restoration most three- and four-hair follicular unit grafts are divided into smaller grafts, this increases the total lifetime donor supply of beard FUE grafts to 8000 to 9000 grafts. Further, many patients will be happy with the results of 2400 to 2700 grafts transplanted in a single day with the option to fill in as needed with a second procedure in 8 months.

Graft harvesting and handling Nearly every beard transplant I perform is done by the FUE rather than the FUT technique. Although most patients are fine with a full shave of the sides and back of the head for facile graft harvesting, some patients prefer modified shaving including a partial-shave FUE (just the lower back of the head) or a no-shave FUE (only the hairs to be extracted are trimmed). These latter approaches present increasing levels of difficulty in harvesting but allow for patients to be presentable faster. For donor-area preparation 2% lidocaine is infiltrated, followed by a tumescent solution of bupivacaine, lidocaine, epinephrine, and triamcinolone in a saline base, providing prolonged anesthesia and reduced bleeding. Sedation with oral medications including diazepam and zolpidem can be complemented by ProNox nitrous oxide during injection.

Our choice of FUE harvesting systems is a hand-held drill that uses an oscillating (rather than rotary) motion. A hybrid punch has a fluted sharp outer edge and only the smooth inner punch surface contacts the hair follicle. The result is a lower rate of transection and the ability to use a smaller punch, usually 0.85 mm. In a typical case, the first 1800 to 2000 grafts are harvested from the back of the head with the patient prone, followed by rotation to supine position with the head tilted slightly back to allow for recipient site formation and graft placement. The grafts are separated, as previously noted, into one- and two-hair grafts, and very importantly the excess skin surrounding the hair follicles is trimmed while leaving the small cuff of fat around the follicles. Excising the excess cuff of skin is the single most important factor in reducing the risk of scarring with tiny bump formation around the grafts, particularly those placed into the chin mound and "soul patch" regions under the central portion of the lower lip. Maintaining graft moisture throughout is critical for reliable regrowth.

Recipient Site Formation and Graft Placement

In most cases, the goatee region is the first area approached for three reasons: first, the donor hairs from the back of the head tend to be the best color

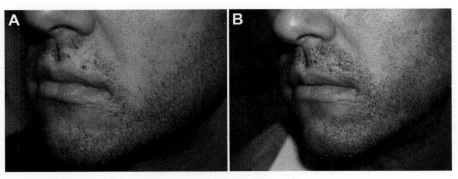

Fig. 4. Facial scar repair, before (*A*) and 1 year after (*B*) 600 FUE grafts.

Table 1
Minimal and maximal graft counts indicated for restoring areas of the beard

Anatomic Area	Minimal Graft Counts	Maximal Graft Counts
Mustache	200	450
Entire goatee (incl mustache)	450	1200
Cheek beard (per side/total)	350/700	900/1800
Sideburns (per side/total)	100/200	300/600

and texture match to those beard hairs in this region; second, this area tends to be the most important, so starting in this area first allows for full attention to restoring; and third, anesthesia in the perioral region is best achieved with nerve blocks of the infraorbital and mental nerves, and this prolonged anesthesia will start to dissipate after 4 to 6 hours coinciding with the patient's lunch break. Supplementing the nerve blocks, small amounts of 2% lidocaine with 1:50,000 epinephrine for prolonged anesthesia and sufficient vasoconstriction are directly infiltrated. Later in the morning and continuing through the rest of the day, once the goatee region has largely been filled, the anesthesia can be extended out laterally into the cheeks and sideburns to allow these areas to be planted. In the posterior cheeks and sideburns, most of the grafts can be those harvested from the sides of the head, as their color and texture are a closer match. In addition, these hairs that are planted later in the day have likewise been harvested later in the day, theoretically improving regrowth.

The occasional patient, particularly in smaller cases, desires the use of beard rather than scalp donor hairs. Beard donor hairs can grow quite reliably and seem natural in the beard.[2] Although it is my experience that scalp hairs yield perfectly natural appearances when transplanted into the beard, the occasional patient insists that only beard donor hairs will be suitable. As long as the patient has enough donor hairs in what is typically the portion of the beard below the lower border of the mandible extending into the upper neck, these hairs can in fact be used instead of or as a supplement to scalp as donor material. Patients are advised that beard donor hairs have a slight risk of a lower percentage of regrowth, but note that in most cases regrowth rates approach that of the gold-standard scalp donor hairs.

Once anesthesia has been obtained, recipient sites are made using most commonly a 0.5-mm

beaver-type blade that we cut ourselves from sharp single-edged razor blades. In nearly all cases, 0.5-mm incisions are appropriate for one- and two-hair graft insertion. This is the key aesthetic step in the transplantation process, for these recipient sites, made by the surgeon, determine hair angulation, direction, distribution, and density. The recipient sites should typically be made as acutely flat to the facial skin as possible, following natural hair growth direction, which changes depending on the anatomic part of the beard. To permit the surgeon full control of where individual grafts get placed, it is best that the surgeon first make most of the two-hair (and if appropriate, three-hair) recipient sites to then be filled by the appropriate grafts, repeating this over several passes until the desired density is achieved, followed then by the surgeon making one-hair recipient sites in between the two-hair grafts as well as along the borders of the restoration to achieve feathering and the ideal naturalness.

For the most expeditious graft planting with least graft trauma, dull implanters are used to insert each graft. This graft placement process is achieved by one team of four assistants, with two loading the implanters one graft at a time and handing this off to the two more experienced assistants who then insert the grafts into the recipient sites. The grafts must be kept moist to avoid desiccation and be gently placed to avoid damage. With this four-person team, it is possible to place 600 grafts per hour.

Graft placement continues with these repeated cycles until all recipient sites are filled. Toward the end of the case, the patient is given the opportunity to observe the restoration and provide feedback, assuring the desired look is achieved. Although there is not uncommonly moderate swelling, the patient and surgeon can largely assess symmetry and overall appearance. Once the procedure is completed, a 4- to 10-hour process, antibiotic ointment is applied to the donor area while the grafted beard is cleaned but left dry.

After the procedure the transplanted areas are to be kept absolutely dry for the first 5 days, whereas normal scalp washing is permitted. On day six, normal face washing can proceed, helping to accelerate the falling off of the tiny crusts, a process that is usually completed at 9 to 10 days, at which point shaving can be resumed. The scalp donor area where FUE was performed is typically healed in 3 days. Normal exercise and activity can be resumed on day six. Most, if not all, of the transplanted hairs will fall off by 2 weeks, with the patient returning to essentially the same appearance as before surgery. Any prolonged erythema can be treated with oral antihistamines or, if

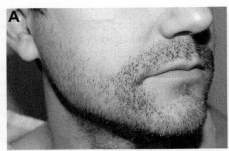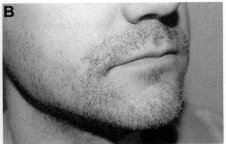

Fig. 5. Reparative beard transplant case, before (*A*) and 3 months after (*B*) FUE removal of 500 prior placed unaesthetic beard grafts primarily around the mustache, then replanted into adjacent areas.

indicated, a course of antibiotics or oral steroids. Regrowth of the transplants starts by 3 to 4 months, and by 8 to 10 months the final result is largely achieved. At this time, if more coverage is desired a second procedure can be performed.

Reparative Beard Transplantation

An unfortunate sequela of the growth in popularity of beard restoration is the increase in patients with unnatural appearances. Most commonly patients are disappointed because of improper hair growth direction that is not sufficiently acute or the use of hair grafts containing three or more hairs. Other reasons for disappointment are unaesthetic beard design, "row" appearance of grafts, and bumps at the base of the hairs most commonly in the chin mound but that can occur anywhere in the beard.

Fortunately, in most cases these appearances can be repaired. Laser hair removal is not the repair procedure of choice due to two limitations: first, it destroys the hairs rather than allowing them to be recycled by being planted either back into the beard or the donor-site scars, and second, it does not usually improve whatever skin scarring exists. Rather, FUE is the preferred method for repairing prior beard transplants, with each prior-placed graft extracted one at a time, using refined FUE techniques, and ultimately minimizing surrounding scarring, as shown in **Figs. 5** and **6**. In nearly all cases, a 0.85-mm punch can fully extract each prior

graft and the small surrounding cuff of skin that often contains scar tissue. Once extracted, these grafts can then be dissected down into one- and two-hair grafts with their excess skin excised, then replanted either into adjacent areas of the beard into newly made recipient sites or returned to the donor-area scars.

Care for these FUE removal sites involves the application of antibiotic ointment for the first 3 days. Normal face washing can be resumed on the second day unless grafts were placed back into the beard in which case dry-face precautions are followed for the first 5 days. Healing is typically rapid with these FUE removal procedures, with most patients having at most only minimal pink dots after 3 days. If a subsequent beard transplant is desired, it can be performed as soon as 6 weeks later.

Body Hair Transplantation (Beard-To-Scalp Transplantation)

BHT has grown tremendously in the field of hair restoration because it overcomes the limited supply/high demand paradigm of hair restoration. In BHT for beard to scalp, beard hairs are extracted by FUE and transplanted into the scalp. Far and away the most common indications for beard-to-scalp transplantation are in cases of advanced degrees of scalp hair loss where patients desire maximal coverage and in reparative cases where

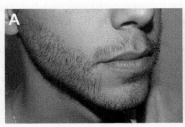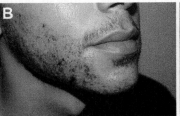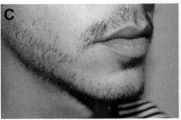

Fig. 6. Reparative beard transplant case, before (*A*), 1 day after (*B*), and 8 months after (*C*) FUE removal of 800 prior placed unaesthetic beard grafts, then replanted into adjacent areas.

Table 2
Total donor supply of the beard (graft numbers) that can be harvested over two to three procedures

Anatomic Area	Minimal Detectable Thinning	Maximal Harvesting
Below the jawline	800–1000	1500–1800
Cheek beard (both sides)	1000–1200	3000–3500
Goatee including mustache	200–400	1000–1500

prior hair transplant procedures, whether FUT or FUE, have partially or nearly completely depleted scalp-hair donor supply.

The beard area contains a large quantity of potential donor hairs. The actual number is determined by the size and the concentration of hairs in the beard and limited by the number of areas the patient will accept having thinned out. **Table 2** summarizes the approximate quantity of hairs that can be harvested from a given area in a typical patient. Note that this table shows two variants—minimal to undetectable thinning and near to total removal of all the hairs in the area.

It is uncommon for most patients to be willing to lose their entire beard. Most prefer to add 800 to 1000 beard grafts to the maximal number of scalp hair grafts of 2400 to 2800 that can be harvested in a single procedure, thus increasing the total graft count by 30% to 40%. These beard hairs will most commonly come from the portions of the beard in the upper neck and below the jawline, essentially leaving no detectability that these hairs were harvested while providing a significant greater amount of scalp coverage (**Fig. 7**). There are, however, some patients, including male-to-female gender reassignment patients and older men, who are motivated to have as many as 3500 grafts removed from the beard in a single procedure to achieve maximal scalp coverage in addition to the available scalp hairs (**Fig. 8**). Even with these large graft extraction numbers, there is essentially no visible scarring of the beard region, with a small risk of

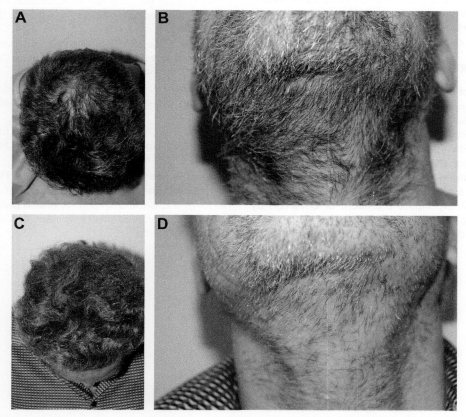

Fig. 7. BHT case, before (*A, B*) and 10 months after (*C, D*) the transplanting of 1600 beard donor hair grafts from below the jawline into the scalp in a case of depleted scalp donor hair supply due to prior procedures.

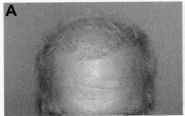 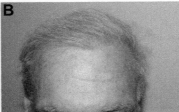 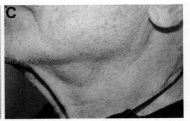

Fig. 8. BHT case, before (*A*) and 1 year after (*B, C*) the transplanting of 3800 beard donor hair grafts into the scalp in a case of depleted scalp donor hair supply due to prior procedures.

delayed healing of the chin mound. Thus, this area should be an area of last choice.

Beard donor hairs have a high reliability of regrowth, coming close to that of scalp hair. Once transplanted, like scalp donor hairs they fall out, start to regrow in 4 months, and then continue to grow as long as scalp hairs, despite having a somewhat different anagen-telogen growth cycle.[8] Typically, these beard hairs will retain their thickness, which is almost twice the shaft caliber of scalp hair, whereas almost all are in one-hair follicular units[8]—an advantage as they provide more coverage—while they tend to lose their coarseness, which in turn improves patient acceptance. The beard donor area is healed in 24 hours, with no detectability as soon as the very next day after the procedure.

SUMMARY

The role of beard hairs in the field of hair restoration surgery is a vital one. Beard transplants permit the creation of more masculine appearances, where transplanting of scalp hairs to the beard can provide natural appearances, even permitting patients to shave without any visible scarring. BHT, involving beard donor hairs for restoring the scalp, is a growing technique in hair restoration surgery. It expands the amount of coverage by expanding the total scalp donor supply achievable in cases of male pattern hair loss as well as in reparative scalp hair transplants when prior procedures have largely exhausted the scalp donor supply.

REFERENCES

1. Gandelman M, Epstein J. Hair transplantation to the eyebrow, eyelashes, and other parts of the body. Facial Plast Surg Clin North Am 2004;12:253–61.
2. True RH. Using nonscalp hair in scalp hair restoration-theory and execution. Ind J Plas Sur 2021;54(4): 463–70.
3. Anastassakis K. Androgenetic alopecia from A to Z. In: Chapter 94: body hair transplantation FUE (BHT FUE)3, 1st edition. Switzerland: Springer; 2023. p. 151–67.
4. Epstein J, Bared A, Kuka G. Ethnic considerations in hair restoration surgery. Facial Plast Surg Clin North Am 2014;22:427–37.
5. Franbourg A, Hallegot P, Baltenneck F, et al. Current research on ethnic hair. J Am Acad Dermatol 2003; 48(6):115–9.
6. Bared A, Epstein J. Gender-affirmation hair transplantation techniques. Facial Plast Surg Clin North Am 2023;31:375–80.
7. Bared A. Beard hair transplantation. Facial Plast Surg Clin North Am 2020;28:237–41.
8. Tolgyesi E, Coble DW, Fang FS, et al. A comparative study of beard and scalp hair. J Soc Cosmet Chem 1983;34:361–82.

Updated Review of Treatment of Androgenetic Alopecia

Roy Xiao, MD, MS[a,b], Linda N. Lee, MD[a,b,c],*

KEYWORDS

- Alopecia • Hair loss • Hair transplant • Quality of life

KEY POINTS

- Alopecia is a common problem affecting men and women. Androgenetic alopecia is the most common form, although hair loss can be multifactorial and deserves comprehensive workup in the appropriate patient.
- Finasteride and minoxidil are the two Food and Drug Administration–approved medical therapies for hair loss that can help stabilize or in certain cases even improve scalp coverage. Platelet-rich plasma is also available for off-label treatment of alopecia with positive outcomes.
- Hair transplantation is an effective therapy using healthy follicular units to reestablish the hair-bearing scalp in appropriately selected patients.

INTRODUCTION

Androgenetic alopecia (AGA) is the most common form of hair loss affecting both men and women.[1,2] It is characterized by progressive hair loss from the scalp that varies in severity, age of onset, and scalp location. Men typically experience hair loss in the vertex and frontotemporal regions with patterns described by the Norwood classification.[3] The prevalence of AGA increases with age, although there is no significant evidence to suggest environmental influence on AGA other than perhaps nicotine exposure.[4,5] That being said, a healthy lifestyle free of stress may affect the epigenetic issues with hair loss.[6] Fundamentally, AGA is polygenetic in nature, and although the exact molecular mechanisms behind AGA remain unknown, androgens (specifically, testosterone and dihydrotestosterone [DHT]) are believed to shorten the anagen (growth phase) in the normal hair growth cycle, resulting in thinner and shorter follicles.[7]

Although hair loss may not cause physical or physiologic harm, a wide range of studies have demonstrated its significant adverse psychosocial impact on patients. Although affected women do report greater psychological harm than men, patients more broadly experience significantly impaired quality of life due to alopecia.[8] Alopecia has also been found to have a significant negative influence on health utility in both sexes.[9] Studies have also found impaired emotions for patients with hair loss but no association with depression.[10]

There are a range of options available to treat patients with hair loss.[11,12] Currently, there are two Food and Drug Administration (FDA)–approved medications for androgenetic alopecia: finasteride and minoxidil. Finasteride acts as a competitive inhibitor of type 2 5α-reductase to inhibit the conversion of testosterone to DHT.[13] Finasteride rapidly lowers serum and scalp DHT levels by greater than 60%, and multiple randomized placebo-controlled studies have demonstrated significantly

[a] Department of Otolaryngology, Massachusetts Eye and Ear, Boston, MA, USA; [b] Department of Otolaryngology, Harvard Medical School, Boston, MA, USA; [c] Division of Facial Plastic and Reconstructive Surgery, Massachusetts Eye and Ear, Boston, MA, USA
* Corresponding author. Division of Facial Plastic and Reconstructive Surgery, Department of Otolaryngology - Head and Neck Surgery, Massachusetts Eye and Ear, 243 Charles Street, Boston, MA 02114.
E-mail address: linda_lee@meei.harvard.edu

Facial Plast Surg Clin N Am 32 (2024) 417–423
https://doi.org/10.1016/j.fsc.2024.02.006
1064-7406/24/© 2024 Elsevier Inc. All rights reserved.

increased hair counts and improved scalp coverage.[14–16] Minoxidil, initially used orally as a potassium channel opener and vasodilator for treatment of hypertension, can be applied topically to stimulate hair growth presumably by extending the duration of anagen to enlarge follicles.[17,18] Oral minoxidil has also shown efficacy for patients with AGA, although its use remains off-label.[19,20] Separately, the Lasercomb (Lasercomb, Notzingen, Germany) is a low-level laser device approved by the FDA to treat alopecia with statistically significant increase in hair density.[21]

Patients may seek more significant improvements in their AGA hair loss beyond the limitations of medical therapies. This may be the case especially when the extent of hair loss begins to affect quality of life. These patients may turn to hair transplantation in which healthy hair follicles are removed from the nonbalding occipital scalp unaffected by androgenic alopecia and transplanted into affected areas.[22,23] These transplanted hair follicles retain their original properties; thus, they are considered permanent compared with the affected areas, although ongoing medical therapies can be critical to maintain the scalp.

Follicular unit grafting has been shown to be highly effective in producing excellent results and high patient satisfaction among men with alopecia.[24] Patients have been found to benefit significantly from hair restoration.[25] Men receiving hair transplantation were found to be perceived as younger, more attractive, more successful, and more approachable according to casual observers.[26] Men with alopecia have been found to have significantly improved self-esteem levels and increased satisfaction with appearance following hair transplantation.[27] Moreover, these patients have been found to have significantly improved perceived health utility following hair transplantation.[9,28]

PATIENT ASSESSMENT

Patients with alopecia can require appropriate diagnostic workup to address potential underlying causes of hair loss and select proper treatment.[29] This workup includes comprehensive history and physical examination, with consideration of differential diagnosis. Slight recession of the hairline is normal in early adulthood with up to 2 cm of posterior recession of the hairline's leading edge.[30] Important alternatives to AGA that must be considered when assessing patients with alopecia include alopecia areata,[31] an immune-mediated form of nonscarring hair loss, traction alopecia resulting from repeated or prolonged tension on hair,[32] cicatricial (scarring) alopecia resulting from infectious or inflammatory conditions,[33] and trichotillomania

that is a psychiatric disorder characterized by recurring hair pulling.[34]

Moreover, vertex and frontal hair loss have been associated with increased rates of cardiovascular disease,[35] as have early-onset hair loss and rapidly progressive hair loss.[36,37] Of note, AGA has also been found to be related to medical conditions including hypertension,[38] obesity,[39] insulin resistance,[40] and even death.[41] Thus, patients with especially early or atypical presentations would benefit from appropriate medical workup.

FOLLICULAR UNIT TRANSPLANTATION

Hair transplantation can provide relatively permanent improvement in androgenetic alopecia using follicular units from the nonbalding occipital scalp.[22] These hair follicles are understood to maintain the characteristics of the occipital scalp donor site that are relatively resistant to AGA; thus, transplanted hair maintains its larger caliber. Two primary techniques are used for modern day hair transplantation: follicular unit transplantation (FUT) and follicular unit excision (FUE). Advancements in our understanding of follicular unit anatomy have enabled modern hair transplantation techniques. Estimates have shown an average of 100 follicular units per square centimeter, with each unit including 2 to 4 terminal follicles and 1 to 2 vellus follicles (thinner hair).[42]

FUT is defined by harvest of occipital scalp tissue, typically as a strip, microscopically dissecting the individual follicular units and reimplanting these units into the recipient sites.[43,44] As such, the donor area must be carefully scrutinized before surgery to understand the number of hairs per surface unit, density of hairs per follicular unit, color and texture of the hair and skin, and laxity and thickness of the scalp.[44] Understanding each of these variables allows for proper preoperative planning to determine the width and overall size of the donor strip to harvest the number of hairs desired for transplant. For most men, there are approximately 6000 to 10,000 hairs available for use from the occipital hairs.[45]

The donor strip is prepared by clipping the site with electric hair clippers to define the region to be harvested.[44] Care is taken to leave hair immediately above and below the strip for postoperative coverage of the wound. Common landmarks to define the limits of the donor site include the horizontal line corresponding to maximum skull circumference superiorly, the occipital protuberance inferiorly, and the ears on each side.[46] The width is typically 10 to 15 mm but can extend up to 20 mm for larger cases if allowed by sufficient skin laxity. Surgeons should avoid the temptation to harvest a wider strip than the skin laxity allows, as visible scarring may result from excessive wound tension. If only a small number of grafts is needed, grafts can be preferentially harvested from the side of the scalp contralateral to how the patient sleeps. In all cases, hair that is not being harvested should not be dissected to preserve them for future transplant.

The surgical site is next anesthetized, typically with 1% lidocaine with 1:100,000 epinephrine, and many surgeons augment this with bupivacaine with 1:100,000 epinephrine.[47] Tranexamic acid can also be included within the tumescent anesthetic to decrease bleeding by inhibiting fibrinolysis.[48] Once appropriate anesthesia has been achieved, a scalpel is used to incise the skin, taking care to angle the blade parallel to the direction of the surrounding follicles to avoid inadvertent transection. The subcutaneous plane is next carefully separated with tumescence, and typically without inadvertent entry into a deeper plane, cautery is not needed. When closing the wound, undermining is typically avoided to avoid disrupting neighboring scalp tissue and causing scar that could affect future transplantations; moreover, there is typically sufficient laxity in the native scalp tissues to allow for closure without much difficulty.

Once the donor strip has been harvested, the hair is next managed by the hair technologists' team assisting the surgeon. The strip is slivered and then carefully prepared into follicular unit grafts of various sizes from usually one to four hairs per graft.

While the grafts are being prepared, the recipient site is prepared. A supraorbital nerve block is used for additional anesthesia followed by injection of the same local anesthetics used in the occipital scalp along the recipient regions. Tranexamic acid can again be included for hemostasis at the recipient site.[49] Typically under magnification (3.5–4.5x), recipient sites are created using either 18-G needles or hair transplant blades customized to the width and depth of the patient's hair. The recipient sites are created to align with the direction of native hairs. Technicians then rapidly place the grafts into the recipient site using fine-tipped forceps. Hair regrowth begins as early as 4 to 6 months postoperatively, and the final result should become evident approximately 1 year after surgery.

FOLLICULAR UNIT EXCISION

In contrast to FUT, FUE involves removal of individual follicular units directly from the donor region of the occipital scalp, sparing the patient a linear harvest scar, but it is important to emphasize it is not entirely scarless, as hypopigmented macules are the norm postoperatively.[50] FUE is performed by individually extracting follicular units from the donor area using a punch measuring 0.7 to 1.0 mm in diameter. FUE was first formally defined and published by Rassman and colleagues in 2002 before subsequent development of more advanced technology and devices capable of assisting surgeons with the procedure.[51] Although harvest was first done using manual sharp punch tools akin to a skin biopsy punch, this has since been replaced with motorized devices. These motorized devices fall into two categories, rotating or oscillating systems, as well as even more modern systems that incorporate multiphasic drill systems that introduce vibration to the dissection process. Modern robotic systems can also be used for extraction.[52] Current commercially available punches fall into three groups: sharp, blunt, or hybrid; sharp punches are more capable of dissecting and accordingly are introduced more superficially to avoid transection of the hairs, whereas blunt punches are introduced deeper and may not cut through the skin as easily, which could cause pressure-related deformities in the hair follicles, if not outright graft burial.

The donor site is prepared differently in FUE compared with FUT.[50] Instead of a donor strip, most often the entire back and sides of the scalp are trimmed using an electric razor while leaving at least 2 mm length to the hairs to discern the natural curve of the hair shaft during FUE. Alternatively, instead of shaving the entire back and sides of the scalp, the bottom 4 to 6 cm along the lower back of the scalp could be selectively trimmed to allow for harvest of up to 1200 to 1400 follicular units. Finally, patients and surgeons could opt for the "no-shave" FUE in which only individual hairs to be extracted are trimmed.[53] "No-shave" FUE could also be performed by extracting the individual follicular units including the entire lengths of the hairs. Regardless of technique, "no-shave" FUE typically increases technical complexity, increases time spent harvesting, and decreases total yield by 10% to 15%.

When planning FUE, surgeons often mark out safe zones intended to be the regions to focus on follicular harvesting.[50] Grafts should be carefully and evenly divided across zones to ensure uniformity, and in the areas surrounding the harvesting region care is taken to create a gradient to ensure no dramatic contrast between densely harvested regions and the neighboring regions. Local anesthesia is similarly achieved using 1% to 2% lidocaine with 1:100,000 epinephrine, and 20 to 25 mL of tumescence is next injected between the subdermal and deep dermal layers to provide sufficient pressure to allow for harvest. Punches are next used, taking care to remain aligned with the directionality of the hair and insert to a depth of no more than 2 to 4 mm depending on the type of punch used. Harvesting is not only a visual exercise but also the experienced practitioner must be able to feel that the graft is not transecting and also feel an appropriate release of the arrector pili muscle/dermis to gauge proper depth.[54] Preparation and insertion of grafts into the recipient site proceed similarly to how they are performed in FUT as described earlier.

Overall, FUE carries the primary benefit of no visible linear scar compared with FUT along with generally shorter and easier recovery period. Moreover, the technique can be used to harvest follicular units from regions of the body other than the scalp, such as hair from the face, chest, or abdomen. However, compared with FUT, FUE typically requires longer operative times to complete extraction (1–2 hours vs 30–45 minutes for FUT), and some surgeons believe that FUE may not yield as many grafts compared with FUT. Moreover, FUE often carries higher costs due to equipment needs and longer case duration. Lastly, excessive harvesting using FUE has been seen to create an iatrogenic "moth-eaten" appearance with visually depleted hair in the donor region.[55]

CONSIDERATIONS IN HAIR TRANSPLANTATION
Patient Selection

Patient selection is critical to ensure success following hair transplantation.[44] Patients with underlying medical conditions or an active scarring process causing the alopecia would likely be poor candidates for hair transplantation and should be counseled accordingly. If a process other than androgenic alopecia is suspected, blood work and a biopsy (in the area of hair loss) should be considered. Moreover, younger patients may present earlier in their hair loss cycle and pose challenges for surgeons, as it can be difficult to predict the extent and pattern of hair loss anticipated for a patient in their early 20s. As such, it would be challenging to create an appropriate new hairline as a younger patient may wish for while native hairs continue to recede. Thus, for such young patients or patients whose hair loss has not stabilized, early focus should be on medical treatment to maintain their hair count and quality until their hair loss is stabilized. More broadly, it is critical to obtain comprehensive photography of the patient from all views including the frontal, three-quarters, profile, occipital, and vertex views.

Gender Considerations

Beard hair transplantation is an increasingly popular technique for natural-appearing facial hair to meet increasing demand from patients.[56,57] Patient goals can vary, although they typically have a clear objective of what they are seeking. Difficulty can range from less challenging cases where patients present with patchiness in existing facial hair seeking increased density to the most challenging cases where patients have essentially no native facial hair. Experts note that it can be less challenging to increase density in the cheek beard rather than the central face, which should be relayed to inform patient decisions. FUE is most often the harvest method of choice for these patients with similar approaches to implantation in the scalp.

Hair transplantation can also serve an important role among a wide range of gender transformation procedures for transgender patients.[58,59] Options include hairline lowering, eyebrow transplantation, and pubic hair transplantation for male-to-female transgender patients and beard and body hair transplantation for female-to-male patients. For these cases, no-shave FUE is oftentimes used to avoid a linear donor site incision and sparing surrounding hairs from being trimmed. Although the surgical technique remains largely the same as what is done in traditional scalp hair transplantation, extra care is required for thoughtful and collaborative preoperative planning, with the patient as part of their transformation. For example, feminizing a hairline typically requires hairline lowering and blunting of the temporal region; subtle details like a slightly off-center widow's peak can help create a more natural-appearing hairline, and rounding of the hairline posteriorly and laterally can help to soften the hairline and achieve greater femininity. It is important to note that hairline lowering and hair transplantation have different risks and different indications, and the distinction is important for patients to understand. Similarly, careful preoperative expectations and design are required for beard and eyebrow transplantation to ensure the locations and shapes of facial hair are consistent with patient desires.

Ethnic Considerations

Special attention must be paid to the unique characteristics and preferences of different patient races and ethnicities when performing hair transplantation.[60,61] For example, Caucasian men typically develop frontotemporal recession, so a conservatively high midpoint and receded frontotemporal angles are recommended to ensure sufficient donor hair to account for further hair loss progression. In contrast, African American men often have no frontotemporal recession, but instead experience a near-straight receding hairline across the forehead. Of note, shaved styles are more common among African American men, so donor strip harvesting in FUT must be carefully considered and discussed with the patient before proceeding, as the scarring pattern may make it difficult to wear such a hairstyle afterward. Asian patients often have rounder and wider heads with a "flat-convex" hairline with less noticeable frontotemporal recession compared with the "round-convex" Caucasian hairline.

COMPLICATIONS OF HAIR TRANSPLANTATION

Like all surgical procedures, FUT can result in complications, although these are rare.[46,62–64] During the procedure itself, and especially while anesthesia is administered, patients can develop anxiety, vasovagal episodes, or even lidocaine toxicity. It is important to calculate the maximum dose of lidocaine allowed for each case based on the patient's weight. Common postoperative issues include bleeding, infection, erythema, swelling, and numbness. Patients can also develop folliculitis, which could require unroofing, although this typically resolves without requiring intervention. Telogen effluvium, or thinning/shedding of hair entering the telogen phase, can also occur following hair transplantation to cause a temporary postoperative hair loss.[65] FUE shares most potential complications with FUT; although, given the inherent approach to FUE, it does carry the risk of unintentional overharvesting, which is permanent.

Most surgeons believe that longer-term complications following hair transplantation are due to errors in surgical planning or execution. Poor patient selection or hairline planning could lead to suboptimal patient outcomes relative to expectations. As mentioned previously, special attention should be paid to ensure no active scarring process occurs in patients receiving hair transplantation.[66] Overall graft survival is typically excellent; however, follicular unit survival has been shown to decrease from approximately 95% following 2-hour processing time to 86% following 6 hours.[67] Thus, graft failure may result secondary to extended transplant time, inadvertent desiccation, graft ischemia, or mechanical damage.[68] Moreover, lichen planopilaris, a type of primary scarring alopecia, has been reported to occur in various degrees of follow-up following hair transplantation, although with unclear association with the procedure itself.[69]

FUTURE DIRECTIONS

PRP has been used across a wide range of applications across facial plastic and reconstructive surgery, including skin rejuvenation (after both resurfacing and microneedling), soft-tissue augmentation, and hair restoration.[70–72] A range of protocols exist for preparing PRP, although traditionally it is centrifuged from 10 to 20 mL of whole blood to separate the red blood cells from the buffy coat containing white blood cells and platelets and plasma above. The plasma and buffy coat are harvested and centrifuged again to produce a platelet pellet, which is resuspended within a lower volume of plasma for a high concentration, which is then used for injection. It is hypothesized to help with AGA by promoting angiogenesis and neocollagenesis through a wide range of growth factors (platelet-derived growth factor, transforming growth factor-beta, vascular endothelial growth factor, and so forth). Although FDA approved in orthopedics, PRP remains off-label use for AGA, although there is an extensive body of research to demonstrate positive outcomes by objective criteria, as well as by patient satisfaction. The only common complications are transient edema or erythema, as well as pain or headache. For AGA, PRP is typically administered in a series of three injections spaced 4 to 6 weeks apart. Similarly, ongoing research continues into alternative cell-based therapies, such as adipose and adipose-derived regenerative cells, which have been shown to increase terminal hair counts in men with early alopecia.[73,74]

SUMMARY

Alopecia is a common problem affecting men and women, and it can cause significant detrimental effects on quality of life. Androgenetic alopecia is the most common form, although hair loss can be multifactorial and may require broader medical workup to assess for underlying causes. Common FDA-approved medical therapies include finasteride and minoxidil, which can help to stabilize hair loss or even improve scalp coverage. Hair transplantation is a highly effective procedure in which healthy follicular units are used to restore the hair-bearing scalp in appropriately selected patients. Experience, sound surgical practice, and appropriate patient expectations are critical to ensure a successful outcome of a typically highly safe and powerful procedure.

REFERENCES

1. Lolli F, Pallotti F, Rossi A, et al. Androgenetic alopecia: a review. Endocrine 2017;57(1):9–17.

2. Sinclair R. Male pattern androgenetic alopecia. BMJ 1998;317(7162):865–9.

3. Norwood OT. Male pattern baldness: classification and incidence. South Med J 1975;68(11):1359–65.

4. Severi G, Sinclair R, Hopper JL, et al. Androgenetic alopecia in men aged 40-69 years: prevalence and risk factors. Br J Dermatol 2003;149(6):1207–13.

5. Kavadya Y, Mysore V. Role of Smoking in Androgenetic Alopecia: A Systematic Review. Int J Trichol 2022;14(2):41–8.

6. Trüeb RM. Understanding Pattern Hair Loss-Hair Biology Impacted by Genes, Androgens, Prostaglandins and Epigenetic Factors. Indian J Plast Surg 2021;54(4):385–92.

7. Hamilton JB. Male hormone stimulation is prerequisite and an incitant in common baldness. Am J Anat 1942;71(3):451–80.

8. Cartwright T, Endean N, Porter A. Illness perceptions, coping and quality of life in patients with alopecia. Br J Dermatol 2009;160(5):1034–9.

9. Abt NB, Quatela O, Heiser A, et al. Association of Hair Loss With Health Utility Measurements Before and After Hair Transplant Surgery in Men and Women. JAMA Facial Plast Surg 2018;20(6):495–500.

10. Huang CH, Fu Y, Chi CC. Health-Related Quality of Life, Depression, and Self-esteem in Patients With Androgenetic Alopecia: A Systematic Review and Meta-analysis. JAMA Dermatol 2021;157(8):963–70.

11. Price VH. Treatment of hair loss. N Engl J Med 1999; 341(13):964–73.

12. Rossi A, Anzalone A, Fortuna MC, et al. Multi-therapies in androgenetic alopecia: review and clinical experiences. Dermatol Ther 2016;29(6):424–32.

13. Rittmaster RS. Finasteride. N Engl J Med 1994; 330(2):120–5.

14. Kaufman KD, Olsen EA, Whiting D, et al. Finasteride in the treatment of men with androgenetic alopecia. Finasteride Male Pattern Hair Loss Study Group. J Am Acad Dermatol 1998;39(4 Pt 1):578–89.

15. Leyden J, Dunlap F, Miller B, et al. Finasteride in the treatment of men with frontal male pattern hair loss. J Am Acad Dermatol 1999;40(6 Pt 1):930–7.

16. Mella JM, Perret MC, Manzotti M, et al. Efficacy and safety of finasteride therapy for androgenetic alopecia: a systematic review. Arch Dermatol 2010; 146(10):1141–50.

17. Buhl AE. Minoxidil's action in hair follicles. J Invest Dermatol 1991;96(5):73S–4S.

18. Katz HI, Hien NT, Prawer SE, et al. Long-term efficacy of topical minoxidil in male pattern baldness. J Am Acad Dermatol 1987;16(3 Pt 2):711–8.

19. Randolph M, Tosti A. Oral minoxidil treatment for hair loss: A review of efficacy and safety. J Am Acad Dermatol 2021;84(3):737–46.

20. Gupta AK, Venkataraman M, Talukder M, et al. Relative Efficacy of Minoxidil and the 5-α Reductase Inhibitors in Androgenetic Alopecia Treatment of Male Patients: A Network Meta-analysis. JAMA Dermatol 2022;158(3):266–74.

21. Jimenez JJ, Wikramanayake TC, Bergfeld W, et al. Efficacy and safety of a low-level laser device in the treatment of male and female pattern hair loss: a multicenter, randomized, sham device-controlled, double-blind study. Am J Clin Dermatol 2014;15(2): 115–27.

22. Avram M, Rogers N. Contemporary hair transplantation. Dermatol Surg 2009;35(11):1705–19.

23. Ishii LE, Lee LN. Hair Transplantation: Advances in Diagnostics, Artistry, and Surgical Techniques. Facial Plast Surg Clin North Am 2020;28(2). xi-xii.

24. Epstein JS. Hair transplantation for men with advanced degrees of hair loss. Plast Reconstr Surg 2003;111(1): 414–21 [discussion 422-4].

25. Epstein J. Benefits of Proper Hair Restoration. JAMA Facial Plast Surg 2016;18(6):419.

26. Bater KL, Ishii M, Joseph A, et al. Perception of Hair Transplant for Androgenetic Alopecia. JAMA Facial Plast Surg 2016;18(6):413–8.

27. Liu F, Miao Y, Li X, et al. The relationship between self-esteem and hair transplantation satisfaction in male androgenetic alopecia patients. J Cosmet Dermatol 2019;18(5):1441–7.

28. Xiao R, Burks CA, Yau J, et al. Health Utility Measures Among Patients with Androgenetic Alopecia After Hair Transplant. Aesthetic Plast Surg 2023;47(2):631–9.

29. Workman K, Piliang M. Approach to the patient with hair loss. J Am Acad Dermatol 2023;89(2S):S3–8.

30. Rassman WR, Pak JP, Kim J. Phenotype of normal hairline maturation. Facial Plast Surg Clin North Am 2013;21(3):317–24.

31. Pratt CH, King LE, Messenger AG, et al. Alopecia areata. Nat Rev Dis Prim 2017;3:17011.

32. Billero V, Miteva M. Traction alopecia: the root of the problem. Clin Cosmet Invest Dermatol 2018;11: 149–59.

33. Headington JT. Cicatricial alopecia. Dermatol Clin 1996;14(4):773–82.

34. Hautmann G, Hercogova J, Lotti T. Trichotillomania. J Am Acad Dermatol 2002;46(6):807–21 [quiz 822-826].

35. Lesko SM, Rosenberg L, Shapiro S. A case-control study of baldness in relation to myocardial infarction in men. JAMA 1993;269(8):998–1003.

36. Schnohr P, Lange P, Nyboe J, et al. Gray hair, baldness, and wrinkles in relation to myocardial infarction: the Copenhagen City Heart Study. Am Heart J 1995;130(5):1003–10.

37. Herrera CR, D'Agostino RB, Gerstman BB, et al. Baldness and coronary heart disease rates in men from the Framingham Study. Am J Epidemiol 1995; 142(8):828–33.

38. Ahouansou S, Le Toumelin P, Crickx B, et al. Association of androgenetic alopecia and hypertension. Eur J Dermatol 2007;17(3):220–2.

39. Hirsso P, Rajala U, Hiltunen L, et al. Obesity and low-grade inflammation among young Finnish men with early-onset alopecia. Dermatology 2007;214(2): 125–9.

40. Matilainen V, Koskela P, Keinänen-Kiukaanniemi S. Early androgenetic alopecia as a marker of insulin resistance. Lancet 2000;356(9236):1165–6.

41. Su LH, Chen LS, Lin SC, et al. Association of androgenetic alopecia with mortality from diabetes mellitus and heart disease. JAMA Dermatol 2013; 149(5):601–6.

42. Headington JT. Transverse microscopic anatomy of the human scalp. A basis for a morphometric approach to disorders of the hair follicle. Arch Dermatol 1984;120(4):449–56.

43. Epstein JS. Follicular-unit hair grafting: state-of-the-art surgical technique. Arch Facial Plast Surg 2003;5(5):439–44.

44. Sand JP. Follicular Unit Transplantation. Facial Plast Surg Clin North Am 2020;28(2):161–7.

45. Nordström REA. "Micrografts" for improvement of the frontal hairline after hair transplantation. Aesthetic Plast Surg 1981;5(1):97–101.

46. Rawnsley JD. Hair restoration. Facial Plast Surg Clin North Am 2008;16(3):289–97.

47. Lam SM. Hair transplant and local anesthetics. Clin Plast Surg 2013;40(4):615–25.

48. Mendieta-Eckert M, Rodero Ortiz R, Rincón Piñeiro R, et al. Tranexamic Acid for Bleeding Control During a Hair Transplant Procedure. Actas Dermosifiliogr 2020;111(5):421–2.

49. Namazi MR. Practice pearl: a novel anesthetic solution for decreasing the blood loss at the recipient site of hair transplantation (Namazi Solution). Aesthetic Plast Surg 2007;31(4):415.

50. Epstein GK, Epstein J, Nikolic J. Follicular Unit Excision: Current Practice and Future Developments. Facial Plast Surg Clin North Am 2020;28(2):169–76.

51. Rassman WR, Bernstein RM, McClellan R, et al. Follicular unit extraction: minimally invasive surgery for hair transplantation. Dermatol Surg 2002;28(8): 720–8.

52. Avram MR, Watkins SA. Robotic follicular unit extraction in hair transplantation. Dermatol Surg 2014; 40(12):1319–27.

53. Harris JA. Follicular unit extraction. Facial Plast Surg Clin North Am 2013;21(3):375–84.

54. Lam SM. Hair transplant 101. St. Louis, MO: Quality Medical Publishing; 2023.

55. Avram MR, Rogers N, Watkins S. Side-effects from follicular unit extraction in hair transplantation. J Cutan Aesthetic Surg 2014;7(3):177–9.

56. Bared A. Beard Hair Transplantation. Facial Plast Surg Clin North Am 2020;28(2):237–41.

57. Epstein J. Facial hair restoration: hair transplantation to eyebrows, beard, sideburns, and eyelashes. Facial Plast Surg Clin North Am 2013;21(3):457–67.

58. Bared A, Epstein JS. Gender-Affirmation Hair Transplantation Techniques. Facial Plast Surg Clin North Am 2023;31(3):375–80.

59. Bared A, Epstein JS. Hair Transplantation Techniques for the Transgender Patient. Facial Plast Surg Clin North Am 2019;27(2):227–32.

60. Epstein J, Bared A, Kuka G. Ethnic considerations in hair restoration surgery. Facial Plast Surg Clin North Am 2014;22(3):427–37.

61. Lam SM, Karamanovski E. Hair restoration in the ethnic patient and review of hair transplant fundamentals. Facial Plast Surg Clin North Am 2010; 18(1):35–42.

62. Lam SM. Complications in hair restoration. Facial Plast Surg Clin North Am 2013;21(4):675–80.

63. Salanitri S, Gonçalves AJ, Helene A, et al. Surgical complications in hair transplantation: a series of 533 procedures. Aesthetic Surg J 2009;29(1):72–6.

64. Nadimi S. Complications with Hair Transplantation. Facial Plast Surg Clin North Am 2020;28(2):225–35.

65. Loh SH, Lew BL, Sim WY. Localized Telogen Effluvium Following Hair Transplantation. Ann Dermatol 2018;30(2):214–7.

66. Lee JA, Levy DA, Patel KG, et al. Hair Transplantation in Frontal Fibrosing Alopecia and Lichen Planopilaris: A Systematic Review. Laryngoscope 2021; 131(1):59–66.

67. Parsley WM, Perez-Meza D. Review of factors affecting the growth and survival of follicular grafts. J Cutan Aesthetic Surg 2010;3(2):69–75.

68. Zhou Y, Zhang J, Yi Y, et al. Characterization and Risk Factors of Folliculitis after Hair Transplantation: A Multicenter Retrospective Study. Plast Reconstr Surg 2023. https://doi.org/10.1097/PRS.000000000 0011175.

69. Donovan J. Lichen planopilaris after hair transplantation: report of 17 cases. Dermatol Surg 2012; 38(12):1998–2004.

70. Sand JP, Nabili V, Kochhar A, et al. Platelet-Rich Plasma for the Aesthetic Surgeon. Facial Plast Surg 2017;33(4):437–43.

71. Chen JX, Justicz N, Lee LN. Platelet-Rich Plasma for the Treatment of Androgenic Alopecia: A Systematic Review. Facial Plast Surg 2018;34(6):631–40.

72. Justicz N, Derakhshan A, Chen JX, et al. Platelet-Rich Plasma for Hair Restoration. Facial Plast Surg Clin North Am 2020;28(2):181–7.

73. Kuka G, Epstein J, Aronowitz J, et al. Cell Enriched Autologous Fat Grafts to Follicular Niche Improves Hair Regrowth in Early Androgenetic Alopecia. Aesthetic Surg J 2020;40(6):NP328–39.

74. Epstein GK, Epstein JS. Mesenchymal Stem Cells and Stromal Vascular Fraction for Hair Loss: Current Status. Facial Plast Surg Clin North Am 2018;26(4): 503–11.

Male Rejuvenation
Injectables

Daniel B. Hall, MD, Leslie R. Kim, MD, MPH*

KEYWORDS

- Male injectables • Male botox • Male fillers • Wrinkles • Contouring
- Male nonsurgical facial rejuvenation • Male aging face

KEY POINTS

- Facial injectables are a nonsurgical option for male facial rejuvenation.
- Botulinum toxin neuromodulation, dermal fillers, and deoxycholic acid can effectively treat the most esthetically concerning areas of the aging face in males.
- Facial injectables differ in treatment location, dosage, and technique in males compared to females.

INTRODUCTION

The popularity of nonsurgical facial rejuvenation among men is dramatically increasing.[1] In a recent survey of 600 injectable-naïve, esthetically oriented men, crow's feet lines (80%), tear troughs (80%), forehead lines (74%), double chin (70%), and glabellar lines (60%) were their top concerns.[2] Injectable treatments offer potential solutions for all of these concerns.

In the United States, botulinum toxin neuromodulation (BoNT) and dermal fillers rank as the most performed nonsurgical cosmetic procedures, totaling over 2.6 million and 1.3 million procedures in 2020, respectively.[3]

This article will review the pharmacology, preparation, pertinent anatomy, technique, risks, and adverse events associated with injectable agents emphasizing unique differences in male anatomy and esthetics.

ANATOMY

Significant soft-tissue variations exist between men and women. Men exhibit more prominent facial expressions and deeper wrinkles due to less subcutaneous fat.[4,5] Additionally, men have denser blood vessels, making them prone to post-injection bruising.[6] Improper use of injectables can lead to feminization of the face, poor cosmetic results, and dissatisfied patients. Understanding these gender-specific differences is vital for safe and effective esthetic procedures.

Neuromodulation

BoNT received Food and Drug Administration (FDA) approval in 2002 as a temporary cosmetic treatment for glabellar frown lines. BoNT is a neurotoxin produced by the bacteria *Clostridium botulinum*. It inhibits acetylcholine release from the presynaptic membrane, resulting in flaccid paralysis of the postsynaptic muscle with a subsequent softening of unwanted facial lines and expressions. Contraindications for BoNT treatment include allergies or hypersensitivity to any of the formulation ingredients (BoNT type A, human albumin). Absolute contraindications for BoNT include neuromuscular and neurodegenerative disorders such as myasthenia gravis. See **Table 1** for a comparison of the FDA-approved BoNTs. These products require suspension into a liquid form for injection, typically with bacteriostatic saline due to reduced injection pain. The volume of saline that is used to reconstitute the BoNT generally ranges from 1 to 4 mL per 100U of Botox. Brands of BoNT differ when it comes to unit equivalence, with conversions shown in **Table 1**. For

The Department of Otolaryngology–Head and Neck Surgery at The Ohio State University, 915 Olentangy River Road # 4000, Columbus, OH 43212, USA
* Corresponding author.
E-mail address: leslie.kim@osumc.edu

Facial Plast Surg Clin N Am 32 (2024) 425–435
https://doi.org/10.1016/j.fsc.2024.02.007

Table 1
Available botulinum toxin neuromodulations and their properties

Property	Botox	Dysport	Xeomin	Jeuveau	Daxxify
Active ingredient	Botulinum toxin type A	Botulinum toxin type A	Botulinum toxin type A	Botulinum toxin type A	Botulinum toxin type A
Dose-equivalent units	1	2.5–3	1–1.3	1	2
Onset of action	2–3 d	2–3 d	2–3 d	2–3 d	2–3 d
Duration of effect	3–4 mo	3–4 mo	3–4 mo	3–4 mo	3–6 mo[21]
Approved uses	Various cosmetic and medical indications, including wrinkles and certain medical conditions	Various cosmetic and medical indications, including wrinkles and certain medical conditions	Various cosmetic and medical indications, including wrinkles and certain medical conditions	Cosmetic use for frown lines	Cosmetic use for frown lines, certain medical conditions
Notes	Marketed as the first botulinum toxin type A product	May have a quicker onset of action for some patients	Naked protein so may decrease antibody formation.[22]	Also known as "Newtox"	Also known as "DAXI"

ease of communication, Botox, the first BoNT to receive FDA clearance, will be discussed in terms of unit delivery per clinical indication, and the reader can adjust that unit dose for other brands. Discussion of Botox as a brand is in no way meant to imply preference or recommendation for the reader but simply presented as a shorthand to discuss unit dosing for a clinical indication.

Limited research exists on BoNT in men. Previous studies found women had faster onset and longer treatment effects than men at equal doses.[7] Proposed explanations include increased mass and strength of the male muscles of facial expression.

Forehead

Females often seek a smooth forehead without any static or dynamic rhytids. Conversely, a smooth forehead is not desired or typical for the male esthetic, so treatment goals should not include complete rhytid elimination. Given that the frontalis is the sole brow elevator, injection technique must account for normal flat male brow shape and position at the supraorbital ridge. In women, the lateral frontalis muscle may be left untreated to allow for lateral brow elevation and characteristic arching of the lateral brow. In men, the lateral aspect of the frontalis must be treated as excess lateral frontalis muscle contraction can lead to a feminine peaked brow position or "Spock" deformity.

Careful inspection and treatment of the superior frontalis muscle in men with androgenic alopecia and high hairlines are needed to avoid unnatural movement in the areas of alopecia. Prior to injection of the frontalis muscle of older male patients, examination must include careful inspection of brow position to identify eyebrow ptosis as overtreatment of the frontalis in these men may unmask or exacerbate their brow ptosis and potential visual field deficits. Initial total dosing recommendations for women are 15 units of Botox versus 20 to 30 units for men.

Glabellar lines

The glabellar region is the most motile and emotionally expressive zone in men. Men are more likely to have a "U" or horizontal glabellar wrinkle pattern because of their larger procerus muscle. Dominant corrugator activity leads to the vertical glabellar furrows.

For treatment of glabellar rhytids in men, starting doses are 50% to 100% higher than the FDA-approved 20 units of Botox for females. Males usually begin with 30 to 40 units, potentially titrating up to 80 units depending on duration of effect and improvement in rhytids.

Crow's feet

For crow's feet, or lateral orbital rhytids, most men have a downward fan lateral canthi wrinkle pattern, whereas women typically have either the central, full, or downward fan pattern. This may reflect the greater involvement of the zygomaticus major muscle.

The esthetic goal for males is to preserve the upper periorbital wrinkles while relaxing the central and lower wrinkles. A deep relaxation of the lateral crow's feet creates the impression of an open and trustful gaze, which befits women very well, but the gender-specific "aggressiveness" men seek is lost. This can be accomplished by injecting only the lower lateral orbital rhytids below the intercanthal line. Typical starting doses are 8 to 16 U of Botox per side in women and 12 to 16 U per side in men.

Nose

Chronic nasalis activity can cause "bunny lines," which are downward oblique rhytids overlying the nasal side walls and dorsum. These differ from horizontal lines that run over the nasal dorsum that result from procerus activity. Men typically require a slightly higher dose of BoNT for treatment of bunny lines, a total of 2 to 6 units of Botox. The depressor septi nasi muscle can be injected in the base of the columella with a total of 2 to 4 units of Botox, to improve a mild nasal tip ptosis.

Perioral lines

Perioral lines are created by photoaging and chronic activation of the orbicularis oris muscle. In the perioral area, men typically have shallower wrinkles than women due to the presence of terminal hairs and increased vascularity.[8] Perioral lines are typically treated with fillers and resurfacing; however, modest BoNT can be beneficial in a select group of patients. Typical starting dose is 4 to 10 units of Botox at the vermilion border. Men need to be counseled that treatment can result in a fuller lip, known as a "lip flip."

Marionette lines

Chronic contraction of the depressor anguli oris (DAO) muscle can lead to the development of marionette lines/folds. They are equally common in female and males though potentially less esthetic concerning in males with facial hair. This can be treated with fillers for deeper lines or BoNT injection into the DAO for more subtle changes. 2 to 4 units of Botox can be injected into the DAO, typically 1 cm inferior and lateral to the oral commissure.

Dimpled chin (peau d'orange)

Hyperactivity of the mentalis muscle and loss of collagen and fat can result in dimpling or wrinkling of the chin, often described as "peau d'orange." This is less common and of less esthetic concern in men compared to women. BoNT therapy can be used to soften the appearance of wrinkling using 2 to 6 units of Botox for females and 2 to 10 units for males. Injection should be performed low in the midline or 2 paramedian injections, to prevent inadvertent treatment of the depressor labii inferioris that can cause smile asymmetry and oral incompetence.

Masseter hypertrophy

Masseter hypertrophy, often due to bruxism, can lead to a widened contour of the mandible. Caution is advised in the treatment of masseter hypertrophy in male patients, as this feature may help to masculinize the face. Additionally, the provider must determine if the widening of the mandible is due to masseteric hypertrophy or normal lateral flaring of the mandible seen in males, which can be determined by having the patient bite down and feeling how much muscle hypertrophy versus bone there is in that individual. Recommended starting dosage is 20 to 40 units of Botox per side. In some cases, inadvertent muscle bulging may occur upon clenching after treatment that can be addressed with a few additional units into the area of bulging. Care should be taken to stay behind the anterior border of the masseter, as inadvertent injection of the risorius muscle, which resides about 1 cm anterior to the masseteric border, may cause temporary unwanted facial paresis. Patients should be cautioned on these uncommon but possible outcomes.

Neck—platysmal banding

BoNT for platysmal banding should only be considered in specific patients, including younger individuals with good skin elasticity or postoperative cases with residual banding. The most significant difference between men and women is the increased muscle mass. Dosing for men is typically 10 to 40 units, compared to 10 to 30 total units for women. It is important to emphasize that true flaccid descent of platysmal bands do not respond well to BoNT treatment, which should be assigned to a surgical remedy like rhytidectomy. Only early signs of muscle descent or by contrast hypertrophic dynamic bands that are noted are amenable to therapeutic benefit.

Post-injection management, complications, and follow-up

Patients should be counseled on the risk of mild swelling or bruising that may occur at injection sites. Icing may help reduce these immediate post-injection side effects. Serious and systemic side effects are rare. Follow-up after the initial treatment is generally recommended at 14 days to evaluate for treatment response, side effects, and inadequate treatment that may require "touch-ups." Duration of treatment varies but typically last from 3 to 4 months. Repeat BoNT dosing continues to reduce muscle bulk and improve skin quality where regular intervals may become longer in duration or less important in terms of consistency of that interval. For men, it will take longer to achieve a result that will require less consistent application, but, as mentioned, complete elimination of wrinkles is not the goal so adjusting that interval will be on a patient-by-patient basis.

Dermal Fillers

The aging face is a function of facial volume loss, resulting from a combination of bony resorption, fat repositioning, and tissue laxity. This can result in troughs, hollows, lines, and deep furrows. Injectable fillers can be used to restore and reposition volume and soften deep or fine lines, creating a more youthful esthetic.

Gender-specific filler placement varies. In a single-practice, age-matched case analysis of men and women, filler injection sites in men included 86% cheeks and/or tear troughs, 40% perioral area and/or marionette lines, 26% nasolabial folds, 18% jawline, 14% chin, 9% lips, 7% temples, 4% nose, and 3% forehead.[9]

Fillers have different physicochemical properties in terms of viscosity, elasticity, and plasticity. Product viscosity describes how it flows through the needle, and G prime (G′) describes its stiffness and ability to resist deformation while being injected.[10] Higher G′ fillers add volume effectively, while lower G′ fillers are ideal for fine lines. Higher G′ fillers may be beneficial in men who have thicker epidermis and dermis. See **Table 2** for a comparison of the available dermal fillers.

Temples

In a youthful face, the temple is convex and seamlessly transitions into the zygomatic arch and the lateral orbital rim. In males, the temples tend to be more naturally depressed compared to females. In an analysis of soft-tissue loss using MRI, Wysong and colleagues[11] noted that the temple is the location of the second greatest loss of subcutaneous tissue (23%) in the aging male face.

Augmentation can be accomplished with hyaluronic acid (HA), calcium hydroxyapatite (CaHA), or poly-L-lactic acid (PLLA). Injection technique can include depots of filler in a supraperiosteal layer via needle or cannula. The medial and superoposterior aspects of the temple provide the most benefit esthetically. A treatment volume of 0.5 to

Table 2
Available dermal fillers and their properties

Dermal Filler	Active Ingredient	Duration of Effect	Viscosity (η)	G Prime (G′)	Indication	Properties
Juvéderm Volbella XC	Hyaluronic Acid	6–12 mo	Low	Low	Lip augmentation and perioral lines	Monophasic high hydrophilic glycosaminoglycan
Juvéderm Vollure XC	Hyaluronic Acid	12–18 mo	Moderate	Moderate	Moderate to severe facial wrinkles and folds	Monophasic high hydrophilic glycosaminoglycan
Juvéderm Plus XC	Hyaluronic Acid	6–12 mo	Moderate	Moderate	Deeper facial wrinkles	Monophasic high hydrophilic glycosaminoglycan
Juvéderm Ultra Plus XC	Hyaluronic Acid	9–12 mo	High	Moderate–high	Severe wrinkles and folds	Monophasic high hydrophilic glycosaminoglycan
Juvéderm Voluma XC	Hyaluronic Acid	Up to 2 y	High	Moderate–high	Cheek augmentation	Monophasic high hydrophilic glycosaminoglycan
Juvéderm Volux XC	Hyaluronic Acid	6–12 mo	High	High	Jawline and chin augmentation	Monophasic high hydrophilic glycosaminoglycan
Belotero Balance (+)	Hyaluronic Acid	6–12 mo	Low	Low	Infraorbital hollows	Monophasic high hydrophilic glycosaminoglycan
Restylane Silk	Hyaluronic Acid	6–12 mo	Low	Low	Lip augmentation and perioral lines	Biphasic high hydrophilic glycosaminoglycan
Restylane Kysse	Hyaluronic Acid	6–12 mo	Moderate-low	Moderate-low	Lip augmentation	Biphasic high hydrophilic glycosaminoglycan
Restylane	Hyaluronic Acid	6–12 mo	Moderate	Moderate	Wrinkles, lip enhancement, and facial folds	Biphasic high hydrophilic glycosaminoglycan
Restylane Eyelight	Hyaluronic Acid	6–12 mo	Moderate	Moderate	Infraorbital hollows	Biphasic high hydrophilic glycosaminoglycan

(continued on next page)

Table 2
(continued)

Dermal Filler	Active Ingredient	Duration of Effect	Viscosity (η)	G Prime (G′)	Indication	Properties
Restylane Refyne	Hyaluronic Acid	6–12 mo	Moderate–high	Moderate–high	Moderate facial wrinkles and folds	Biphasic high hydrophilic glycosaminoglycan
Restylane Contour	Hyaluronic Acid	12–18 mo	Moderate–high	High	Facial contouring and restoring volume	Biphasic high hydrophilic glycosaminoglycan
Restylane Defyne	Hyaluronic Acid	6–12 mo	High	High	Deeper/severe wrinkles and folds	Biphasic high hydrophilic glycosaminoglycan
Restylane Lyft	Hyaluronic Acid	6–12 mo	High	High	Cheek augmentation	Biphasic high hydrophilic glycosaminoglycan
Radiesse	Calcium Hydroxyapatite	12–18 mo	High	High	Ideal for deeper wrinkles and facial shaping. Contraindicated in the lips and glabella due to unacceptable rates of nodule formation.[23]	Recruit fibroblasts which secrete new collagen
Sculptra	Poly-ʟ-Lactic Acid	2–5 y	Low	Low	Cheek rhytids, nasolabial folds, and marionette lines. Requires series of injections.	Inert polymer. Stimulate synthesis of collagen, resulting in gradual results over time.
ArteFill	Polymethylmethacrylate (PMMA) microspheres suspended in bovine collagen	Permanent[24]	High	High	Requires skin allergy testing due to collagen suspension.	Non-biodegradable material. Final effect created by 80% neocollagenesis and 20% PMMA.[24]

2.0 mL of dermal filler is recommended and 2 to 3 treatments of PLLA may be required. Inadvertent injection into the superficial temporal artery can result in retrograde flow via arterial anastomoses potentially allowing for embolization into the ophthalmic artery which may cause blindness.

Glabella

Injectable fillers can be used to soften deep static glabellar furrows that do not respond fully to BoNT. Filler injections in the glabella are more common in men than in women, as men often present later than women for esthetic consultation when glabellar rhytids are deeply furrowed. Fillers are ideally injected 2 weeks after neurotoxin has achieved maximal effect, as the use of BoNT and dermal fillers has been shown to be more effective in treating glabellar rhytids than fillers alone.[12]

Low-viscosity fillers, like HA filler, are best suited for glabellar furrows. Injection via cannula is recommended. The injection should be placed in the superficial or mid-dermis below the rhytid to provide volume. Total volume of filler required for volume correction of glabellar rhytids is 0.1 to 0.3 mL per furrow. Care should be taken not to overtreat the male glabellar rhytids as men prefer to have some residual expression as compared to females who prefer a smoother contour.

The glabella is a vascular-rich area with anastomoses between the internal and the external carotid artery systems. There is a higher risk of complication when injecting filler into the glabella, including vascular compression, intravascular injection, tissue necrosis, and blindness due to embolization. Smaller filler volumes with fillers that have lower viscosity are recommended to help prevent irregular contours or compression of vessels. Unfortunately, pulling back on the syringe to evaluate backflow does not eliminate or even diminish the risk of intravascular injection.

Midface

The female cheek is fuller, higher, and more projected in all dimensions. The malar prominence in females has a well-defined apex and is located high on the midface, below and lateral to the lateral canthus. The ratio of medial to lateral cheek volume in females is 1.5:1. Conversely, the male cheek has more anteromedial fullness, a broader based malar prominence, and an apex that is more medial and subtly defined. The frontal and zygomatic processes are wider in males, creating a flatter appearance. The ratio of the medial to lateral cheek in men is ideally 1.1:1.[13] While treating male patients, over projection, excessive height, and fullness of the cheeks must be avoided to prevent feminization.

Because correction of the midface may have an esthetic impact on both the upper and lower face, many providers recommend treating the midface first to create a foundation for the entire face. Higher G′ HA filler and CaHA fillers are bested suite for cheek augmentation, as they provide greater support and lifting capacity. For severe volume loss, a series of PLLA injections over multiple months can help restore volume.

Treatment of the midface should always begin by addressing the lateral lifting vectors along the zygomatic arch. Addressing the lateral cheek primarily may result in less augmentation needed medially. Augmentation can be performed in the deep subcutaneous and supraperiosteal planes using needle or cannula technique, with cannula having less risk of vascular injury. If a cannula is used, no smaller than a 25G should be considered, as smaller cannulas can act like a needle in their ability to puncture a vessel. If submalar augmentation is required, cross-hatching in the subcutaneous or dermal-subcutaneous junction is recommended since there is no bony support. Total volume varies based on the volumetric deficit.

Tear trough deformity

Aging causes descent of the malar fat pad inferiorly and medially, leading to the creation of the tear trough or nasojugal deformity. This occurs more significantly in men compared to women. In an MRI study, men had the greatest loss of soft-tissue thickness in the tear trough (40% reduction) compared to other areas of the face.[11] Additional esthetic concerns may include pseudoherniation of the periorbital fat or attenuated orbicularis muscle and lax skin creating festoons, referred to as malar bags. Care must be taken as dermal fillers may exacerbate their appearance.

In the tear trough region, lower G′ HA filler may prevent uneven contour. Less hydrophilic fillers are preferred to avoid post-injection swelling. Injection technique is best accomplished via cannula, below the orbicularis oculi muscle in a supraperiosteal plane to minimize the risk of vascular injury which can rarely result in blindness. Correct placement may help prevent abnormal contour and Tyndall effect. Total dosage ranges from 0.5 to 1 mL distributed medially, centrally, and laterally. When correcting a tear trough defect, it is often necessary to inject more laterally along the zygomatic arch to give the cheek an inferiomedial apex, which is a characteristic masculine feature. If performing cheek augmentation, this should be done first to avoid overcorrection of the tear trough. Despite the best efforts at tear trough augmentation with HA filler, filler may migrate superficially even years later, especially apparent during smiling. The lesson is that fillers do not simply vanish in a few months to a year but has been shown with MRI to persist for years, if not indefinitely.

Nonsurgical rhinoplasty

The ideal male nose is wider with a straight dorsum and a nasolabial angle of 90° to 95° with less nostril show. Nonsurgical rhinoplasty can include camouflage of a dorsal hump by injecting above and below the hump to smooth the transition. It can also be used to raise the radix and elongate the nose. A wide nasal dorsum or post-surgical open vault can be made to appear narrower with dorsal filler. Alar and tip abnormalities may also be treated with filler, though typically more challenging.

Low G' fillers are preferred due to the thin skin of the nose. Injections can be performed either with a needle or cannula. The filler should be placed in the supraperiosteal or supraperichondrial plane, accordingly, and undercorrection is recommended. Apart from intravascular occlusion, complications can also occur due to excessive volume leading to pressure necrosis. The angular artery at the nasal ala, the supraorbital and supratrochlear arteries superiorly, and the lateral nasal arteries at the lateral nasal walls are at greatest risk.

Nasolabial folds

Prominent nasolabial or melolabial folds result due to midface atrophy and descent associated with aging. Nasolabial folds are equally pronounced in men compared to women.[5] Given that the nasolabial fold is more pronounced with midfacial aging, it is recommended to begin with cheek augmentation before approaching the nasolabial folds.

Filler is typically placed via needle or cannula in the deep dermal or superficial subcutaneous plane within the fold itself or immediately medial. Filler placed lateral to the nasolabial folds will accentuate midface descent and deepen the nasolabial fold. For individuals with a hypoplastic maxilla, periosteal depots with a needle can be performed at the upper aspect of the nasolabial fold. However, given the location of the facial artery and its branches, extreme care must be taken when injecting in this area.

Mild to moderate folds respond best to lower G' HA fillers. More severe folds may respond best to higher G' HA fillers or CaHA products. Men typically require greater volumes compared to women. Typical total dosage per side ranges from 0.3 to 1 mL depending on the severity of the fold. Polymethylmethacrylate fillers may also be effective in men for incremental nasolabial fold softening.

Lips

Labial sexual dimorphism is well reported in the literature. The upper lip is larger than the lower lip in women and older men, while young men have a larger lower lip. In men, the upper lip should have a slightly more anterior projection (1–2 mm) on profile and the volume ratio of upper lip to lower lip should be approximately one-third to two-thirds, respectively. After the fifth decade of life, the lips become smaller and thinner in both sexes.[14] Men are less likely to undergo lip augmentation due to the stigmata and risk of overcorrection and feminization. However, there are male patients who may benefit from lip augmentation; for example, patients' with inturned lips and no vermillion show.

Lip augmentation can be performed via needle and/or cannula delivery in a superficial subcutaneous plane. Since the superior and inferior labial arteries are situated in the deep orbicularis oris muscle adjacent to the vermillion border, filler injections should be performed superficial to the orbicularis oculi muscle. Lower G' HA fillers are recommended for lip augmentation. Avoid excess volume and accentuation of the Cupid's bow and the vermillion border to avoid feminization of the lips.

Marionette lines

Labiomandibular folds extend from the oral commissure down to the mandible and are termed marionette lines. Marionette lines are more pronounced in men compared to women.[5] The treatment of marionette lines is similar to the treatment of the nasolabial folds. Low G' HA fillers are mostly commonly employed to treat marionette lines. Filler is injected beneath the lines or medial to the lines, as lateral injection can increase the appearance of the fold. Needle depots or cannula is recommended in a subdermal plane to fill to correct the volume loss of the groove and lift the oral commissure.

Chin

With aging, a loss of mandibular height and length leads to an obtuse mandibular angle, chin retrusion, and an exaggerated prejowl sulcus. The ideal chin in females is the same width as the medial intercanthal distance. Conversely, men have a wider chin that ideally extends to the oral commissures. There are many guidelines as to the ideal chin projection in an anterior-posterior view.[15] A simple rule is that the ideal male chin should project as far as the lower lip, where the ideal female chin should be 1 to 2 mm behind the lower lip. Finally, chin height is an important variable. Ideally, the upper, middle, and lower thirds of the faces should be equal in height. An alternative method for analyzing chin height is that the distance from the subnasale to the inferior margin of the vermilion of the upper lip should ideally be one-third of the distance from the subnasale to the menton.[15]

Chin augmentation can be accomplished with HA, CaHA, and PLLA fillers. Higher G′ fillers may prove beneficial for chin augmentation due to thicker skin and loss of bony support. Injection technique can include needle depots or cannula technique. Male patients may benefit from augmenting chin width to achieve a more masculine ideal. Injection too far laterally may injure the mental artery and nerve. To augment chin height, filler should be placed at the menton in either a supraperiosteal or subcutaneous plane. In a multicenter study of HA filler for facial rejuvenation, the mean total filler used for chin augmentation was 1.1 mL ± 0.9.[16] A final area of concern may be a deep labiomental sulcus. Filler can be used to soften this crease.

Jawline

In the lower face, age-associated resorption of the mandibular bone and midface atrophy and descent results in a loss of the youthful jawline definition with ptosis of the skin and jowling. The esthetic goal in jawline rejuvenation is to straighten the jawline, smooth the transition between the mentum and the jowls, and lift the jowls upwards and posteriorly.

Significant gender differences must be accounted for. The ideal male jaw is more angular and more prominent compared to women. Ideally, men have a bizygomatic to bigonial distance that is approximately 1:1, where a woman's face is characterized by the inverted "triangle of youth," with a bizygomatic distance that is wider than the bigonial distance. The male mandible is 1 of the most characteristic features of a masculine face. Men also have large masseter muscles, which provide further definition. Prominent angulation of the mandibular ramus is typical of the male jaw. As men age, the mandible becomes longer and wider in shape.

In an age-matched case analysis of injectable filler locations in men and women, male patients outnumbered their female counterparts 6:1 for filler injections along the jawline.[9] Injectable materials can include HA, CaHA, or PLLA. In patients with insufficient bony support, higher G′ fillers may be beneficial. Conversely, patients with a well-defined bony structure with thick or thin skin may benefit from either lower G′ fillers or a combination of lower and higher G′ fillers.

Injection technique involves a combination of supraperiosteal and subcutaneous injection. Augmentation starts at the mandibular angle where a single or a series of needle depots are placed to add length to the mandible. To feminize the jawline, filler is placed subcutaneously in an oblique line from the mandibular angle to the ear lobe using a cannula. Conversely, to masculinize the face, filler is placed superiorly along the mandibular ramus in a subcutaneous plane to create a squarer, more angular appearance. To further widen the male jawline, filler can be placed subcutaneously over the masseter using a cannula to avoid inadvertent injection into the parotid gland or facial vein. Finally, in a subcutaneous plane using a cannula, filler can be placed along the mandibular body to lift the jowl and smooth the transition to the prejowl area. Cannula technique may help reduce the risk of injury to the facial artery. Total starting dosage ranges from 1 to 3 mL of filler per side.

POST-INJECTION MANAGEMENT, COMPLICATIONS, AND FOLLOW-UP

Common filler complications include erythema, ecchymosis, tenderness, pruritus, and edema. These symptoms are typically mild and self-resolving. Other potential complications, albeit rarer, include infection, lumps and nodules, and foreign-body granuloma formation. Antibiotics should be given if there is a concern for infection. Lumps and nodules are self-limited but may be treated with massage, touch-up filler to camouflage, or hyaluronidase injection. Tyndall effect, described as blue scattering of light by the filler when placed superficially under the skin, most commonly occurs in areas of thin skin like the lower eyelid. Hyaluronidase injection can be helpful in degrading HA fillers but may also be beneficial for CaHA fillers.[17] For patients with a history of herpes simplex virus, prophylaxis with an oral antiviral medication should be considered. Lip filler has been shown to have a higher rate of herpetic reactivation.[18] Post-injection herpetic outbreak should be treated promptly.

Rare but significant complications from filler injection include soft-tissue necrosis due to vascular injury or compression along with vision loss. Skin necrosis can occur due to vascular injury, intravascular injection, or vascular compression from excess filler placement. Signs and symptoms that may suggest vascular injury include pain and blanching with a reticulate vascular pattern along the distribution of the artery, changes to vision, and rarely stroke. High-risk areas include the glabella, nasal bridge, and upper nasolabial folds, yet filler-induced vascular injury can occur anywhere on the face.

At the onset of any warning sign of vascular occlusion, the practitioner should immediately infiltrate the area of pending necrosis with injectable hyaluronidase, apply warm compresses, and consider administering aspirin, hyperbaric oxygen, and/or low–molecular weight heparin. Topical nitroglycerin use for vascular injury has been reported but its efficacy is controversial.[19] If there is concern for vision changes or vision loss, immediate ophthalmology consultation, ocular massage, timolol eye drops, diuretics, corticosteroids, calcium channel blockers, anticoagulation, and needle decompression of the anterior chamber should be considered. Prognosis is poor with over 50% of cases resulting in blindness.[20]

An expert knowledge of facial vascular anatomy is essential to safe injection technique. Other safeguards include the use of small-gauge needles to slow the rate and amount of injection, avoiding injecting excess volume into a single area, aspirating prior to injection, the use of cannula technique, and avoiding excess force when injecting.

Deoxycholic Acid

Double chin is 1 of the top concerns among esthetically oriented men.[2] Deoxycholic acid, an injectable surfactant approved for convexity or fullness of submental fat, works by emulsifying adipocyte cell membranes resulting in apoptosis. It has demonstrated safety and efficacy in improving the appearance of a double chin. The reduction of submental fat will not only improve the appearance of the double chin but may also help define the masculine jawline. It is important to note that a more mature neck (over the age of 40 years) with skin laxity may show greater skin laxity and/or exposure of underlying platysmal bands, so caution should be taken for an older patient using deoxycholic acid. In addition, neck fullness can oftentimes be attributed to subplatysmal fullness, in which case deoxycholic acid would have limited benefit.

Deoxycholic acid dosing is largely dependent on the treatment area involved. Since male necks are traditionally larger with more substantial and lateral reaching submental fat than female necks, the treatment dose is generally larger. Superior results in male patients may be achieved with 3 to 6 treatments spaced 6 to 8 weeks apart. Adverse events are rare and include edema, pain, bruising, hyperpigmentation, paresthesias, alopecia, and nodule formation. It is important to note that deoxycholic acid only treats subcutaneous adiposity; therefore, patients with a more significant obtuse cervicomental angle should be evaluated for surgical treatment.

REFERENCES

1. Lem M, Pham JT, Kim JK, et al. Changing aesthetic surgery interest in men: an 18-year analysis. Aesthetic Plast Surg 2023;1–6. https://doi.org/10.1007/s00266-023-03344-9.

2. Jagdeo J, Keaney T, Narurkar V, et al. Facial treatment preferences among aesthetically oriented men. Dermatol Surg 2016;42(10):1155–63.

3. Aesthetic plastic surgery national databank statistics 2020-2021. Aesthetic Surg J 2022;42(Suppl 1):1–18.

4. Weeden JC, Trotman CA, Faraway JJ. Three dimensional analysis of facial movement in normal adults: influence of sex and facial shape. Angle Orthod 2001;71(2):132–40.

5. Tsukahara K, Hotta M, Osanai O, et al. Gender-dependent differences in degree of facial wrinkles. Skin Res Technol 2013;19(1):e65–71.

6. Moretti G, Ellis RA, Mescon H. Vascular patterns in the skin of the face. J Invest Dermatol 1959;33:103–12.

7. Rappl T, Parvizi W, Friedl H, et al. Onset and duration of effect of incobotulinumtoxinA, onabotulinumtoxinA, and abobotulinumtoxinA in the treatment of glabellar frown lines: a randomized, double-blind study. Clin Cosmet Invest Dermatol 2013;211. https://doi.org/10.2147/ccid.s41537.

8. Paes EC, Teepen HJ, Koop WA, et al. Perioral wrinkles: histologic differences between men and women. Aesthetic Surg J 2009;29(6):467–72.

9. Wang JV, Valiga A, Albornoz CA, et al. Comparison of injectable filler locations in men and women: An age-matched case analysis. J Cosmet Dermatol 2021;20(8):2469–71.

10. De La Guardia C, Virno A, Musumeci M, et al. Rheologic and physicochemical characteristics of hyaluronic acid fillers: overview and relationship to product performance. Facial Plast Surg 2022;38(02):116–23.

11. Wysong A, Kim D, Joseph T, et al. Quantifying soft tissue loss in the aging male face using magnetic resonance imaging. Dermatol Surg 2014;40(7):786–93.

12. Carruthers J, Carruthers A. A prospective, randomized, parallel group study analyzing the effect of BTX-A (Botox) and nonanimal sourced hyaluronic acid (NASHA, Restylane) in combination compared with NASHA (Restylane) alone in severe glabellar rhytides in adult female subjects: treatment of severe glabellar rhytides with a hyaluronic acid derivative compared with the derivative and BTX-A. Dermatol Surg 2003;29(8):802–9.

13. Goel A, Rai K. Midface Rejuvenation Using Juvederm Fillers in Male Patients. J Cutan Aesthetic Surg 2022;15(3):209–15.

14. Rohrich RJ, Janis JE, Kenkel JM. Male rhinoplasty. Plast Reconstr Surg 2003;112(4):1071–85. quiz 1086.

15. Sykes JM, Suárez GA. Chin advancement, augmentation, and reduction as adjuncts to rhinoplasty. Clin Plast Surg 2016;43(1):295–306.

16. Talarico S, Meski AP, Buratini L, et al. High patient satisfaction of a hyaluronic acid filler producing enduring full-facial volume restoration: an 18-month open multicenter study. Dermatol Surg 2015; 41(12):1361–9.

17. Daines SM, Williams EF. Complications associated with injectable soft-tissue fillers: a 5-year retrospective review. JAMA Facial Plast Surg 2013;15(3): 226–31.

18. Carruthers J, Klein AW, Carruthers A, et al. Safety and efficacy of nonanimal stabilized hyaluronic acid for improvement of mouth corners. Dermatol Surg 2005;31(3):276–80.

19. Hwang CJ, Morgan PV, Pimentel A, et al. Rethinking the role of nitroglycerin ointment in ischemic vascular filler complications: an animal model with ICG imaging. Ophthalmic Plast Reconstr Surg 2016;32(2): 118–22.

20. Ozturk CN, Li Y, Tung R, et al. Complications following injection of soft-tissue fillers. Aesthetic Surg J 2013;33(6):862–77.

21. Bertucci V, Solish N, Kaufman-Janette J, et al. DaxibotulinumtoxinA for Injection has a prolonged duration of response in the treatment of glabellar lines: Pooled data from two multicenter, randomized, double-blind, placebo-controlled, phase 3 studies (SAKURA 1 and SAKURA 2). J Am Acad Dermatol 2020;82(4):838–45.

22. Lorenc ZP, Kenkel JM, Fagien S, et al. Consensus panel's assessment and recommendations on the use of 3 botulinum toxin type A products in facial aesthetics. Aesthetic Surg J 2013;33(1 Suppl): 35s–40s.

23. Graivier MH, Bass LS, Busso M, et al. Calcium hydroxylapatite (Radiesse) for correction of the mid- and lower face: consensus recommendations. Plast Reconstr Surg 2007;120(6 Suppl):55s–66s.

24. Cohen SR, Berner CF, Busso M, et al. ArteFill: a long-lasting injectable wrinkle filler material–summary of the U.S. Food and Drug Administration trials and a progress report on 4- to 5-year outcomes. Plast Reconstr Surg 2006;118(3 Suppl):64s–76s.

Minimally Invasive Male Facial Rejuvenation
Energy-Based Devices

Michael Somenek, MD

KEYWORDS

- Energy based devices • Male plastic surgery • Laser resurfacing • Skin rejuvenation

KEY POINTS

- The development of minimally invasive, non-surgical, and office-based procedures that have minimal downtime has stimulated an interest among men who may seek cosmetic treatments to increase competitiveness and appear youthful in the workplace.
- Male skin has some notable differences compared to female skin that can impact its care and maintenance.
- A variety of energy-based devices exist to treat the common skin conditions that males seek to improve.

INTRODUCTION

Men are an increasingly fast-growing segment of the cosmetic surgery population, representing 10% of all cosmetic procedures performed in the United States (US) each year.

According to a 2020 American Society of Plastic Surgeons statistics report, the number of minimally invasive cosmetic procedures has increased by 72% since 2000. The most popular non-surgical facial procedures include botulinum toxin injections, soft-tissue fillers, laser skin resurfacing, and chemical peels.[1]

There are certain psychologic and social factors that have motivated men to pursue such treatments. In the 1980s, there was a shift of how the male body was objectified, which began to diffuse into popular culture. The commercialization of masculinity coincided with a surge in lifestyle magazines, television, and movies promoting men's fashions and other products. This trend has continued and is a driving force for the male cosmetic industry.[2]

The development of minimally invasive, non-surgical, and office-based procedures (**Table 1**)

that have minimal downtime has stimulated an interest among men who may seek cosmetic treatments to increase competitiveness and appear youthful in the workplace. There has also been greater media attention on the male appearance and grooming along with increasing acceptance of cosmetic procedures within society.[3,4]

Achieving a successful cosmetic treatment in a male patient requires the physician to recognize the gender differences that exist. These include anatomy, skin aging, and skin biology, as well as behavioral patterns that exist in this population.

Male Skin

While the fundamental structure and function of human skin are similar between males and females, there are some notable differences in male skin that can impact its care and maintenance. These differences are primarily influenced by hormonal variations and lifestyle factors.

Male skin produces more sebaceous, eccrine, and apocrine secretions than female skin due to higher levels of testosterone, which can lead to increased sebum production. This may make

Somenek+Pittman MD, Advanced Plastic Surgery, 2440 M Street NW, Suite 507, Washington, DC 20037, USA
E-mail address: Drsomenek@spmeddc.com

Facial Plast Surg Clin N Am 32 (2024) 437–445
https://doi.org/10.1016/j.fsc.2024.03.001

Table 1
Energy based skin treatments

Intense Pulsed Light	Solar Lentignes, Rosacea, and Telangiectasias
RF Microneedling RF Monopolar RF	Skin texture, pores, skin tightening
Ablative resurfacing CO_2 Erbium:YAG	Skin resurfacing
Nd:YAG	Telangiectasias, rosacea, and laser hair removal

Abbreviations: RF, radiofrequency; Erbium:YAG, erbium-doped yttrium aluminum garnet; Nd:YAG, neodymium-doped yttrium aluminum.

male skin more prone to acne and oily skin compared to female skin. The sebaceous glands are larger and more abundant in male skin, especially on the face because they are tied to terminal hairs instead of the vellus hairs characteristic of the female face.

Testosterone can also affect the aging process. Men tend to experience a slower rate of collagen loss, which means that signs of aging, such as wrinkles and sagging skin, may appear later than in women. However, when signs of aging do appear, they can be more pronounced in men.

Male skin functions differently than female skin with respect to skin moisturization needs. Transepidermal water loss (TEWL) is used to assess skin water barrier function.[5] Luebberding and colleagues showed that in participants aged less than 50 years, TEWL in men was significantly lower than in women of the same age, regardless of the location. In participants aged 50 to 60 years, TEWL on the forehead, cheeks, and neck in men was higher than in women of the same age. In most sites, water loss was stable or increased over subjects' lifetime in both sexes. Even though males have increased sebum production, as they age their ability to maintain skin hydration decreases and reinforces the need for a comprehensive skincare regimen and moisturizer.[6]

Male skin is generally thicker than female skin. This increased thickness is primarily due to a higher density of collagen and elastin fibers. As a result, male skin may appear firmer and more resilient. In 1975, Shuster and colleagues first demonstrated that skin thickness in men decreased linearly with age, starting at age 20 years. However, skin thickness remained constant in women until the age of approximately 50 years, at which time skin thickness started decreasing.[7]

There are significant differences in hair distribution in males compared to female skin. Men have more facial hair than women largely due to the effects that androgens have on hair growth. While women have some facial hair, it is usually not as thick or coarse as in men. Men's skin is about 25% thicker than in women with a thicker dermal component, whereas female facial skin shows more subcutaneous fat than in males.[8] Despite the increased thickness in male skin, it can be more sensitive due to a number of factors. The majority of the general population assess themselves as having sensitive skin.[9] Although this is considered to be a more prevalent problem for women, the number of men claiming to have sensitive skin is substantial. Shaving can largely contribute to the overall sensitivity and skin irritation depending on the thickness, coarseness, and density of the facial hair. This is something to keep in mind when recommending skin treatments and procedures that may require abstaining from shaving due to the effects it may have on overall healing and skin irritation.

Wrinkle formation tends to be more severe and develop at an earlier age in men. There are several factors that contribute to skin wrinkles including dynamic facial muscle contraction, oxidative stress, and ultraviolet (UV) radiation.[10] The forehead seems to be the first place for severe wrinkle formation in men in contrast to the periorbital lines in women. Although the development of facial wrinkles happens earlier and is more severe in men, perimenopause seems to particularly affect development in women.[11] The periorbital region has variations that exist with regards to specific patterns of muscle movement and crow's feet formation. Relationships between gender and crow's feet lines show that males predominantly exhibited lower fan movement with wrinkling in both the lower lid and upper cheek area. This is contrast to females, which commonly exhibit a full fan (crinkling of lateral canthal skin from lower lateral brow, through the lateral canthus, and across the lower eyelid/upper cheek junction) or central fan pattern (severe wrinkles only in the skin immediately surrounding the lateral canthus). The variability of the fan pattern can have implications that are specific to neuromodulators.[12] The differences in male skin compared to female skin have been summarized in **Box 1**.

Extrinsic Factors

There are several extrinsic factors that exist, which contribute to some variations in how male skin ages. Men have consistently underutilized preventive health care services including dermatologic care compared with women.[13]

Smoking causes cutaneous injury by decreasing capillary flow to the skin. Nearly 1 in 4 adults in the world smokes tobacco, but there are large differences between men and women. More than one-third of men in the world smoke whereas less than 1 in 10 women do.[14,15] A dose-response relationship between wrinkling and smoking has been identified in addition to increased incidence of facial elastosis and telangiectasia formation among men. Ultraviolet light exposure accelerates cutaneous aging through the degradation of the collagen matrix. Due to the highly gendered nature of employment, men are more likely to be exposed to UV light exposure through outdoor occupations. Additionally, men are less likely to use sun protective behaviors. In a study to assess men's motivations and behaviors toward daily skincare use, it was found that 83% of the study population reported not using sunscreen daily.[16] Another study found that men exhibited a significantly higher frequency of sunburn, employed fewer sun-protective measures, and demonstrated less knowledge concerning sun safety information and skin cancer than women.[17]

Energy-based devices
Intense pulsed light Intense pulsed light (IPL) is a non-ablative fractional laser therapy in which fragmental thermal damage is induced within the exposed skin. Intense pulsed light emits polychromatic light across a broad wavelength spectrum making it fundamentally different from a laser. The broad spectrum provides greater versatility in treating many skin types and conditions.

Intense pulsed light is able to penetrate the tissues, and depending on the selected wavelength, can be absorbed by melanin and hemoglobin, thereby producing photothermal effects. This can be an extremely effective treatment for solar lentigines, telangiectasias, and generalized erythema.[18] Due to the numerous extrinsic factors contributing to the changes in aging male skin,

this can provide a simple, low downtime solution to many concerns that males have with their skin appearance. Due to the increased thickness of male skin, men may need more treatments, and higher energy settings than women to achieve satisfactory results.

Rosacea is a chronic cutaneous disorder primarily affecting the face. It is characterized by erythema that may be transient or persistent, telangiectasias, and possible papulo-pustules. It affects up to 10% of the world's population with women being more affected than men.[19] However, rhinophyma, which is the final and most severe stage of rosacea, primarily affects white males over the age of 50. Men have a higher density of facial blood vessels than women, and they often seek treatment for telangiectasias and overall facial erythema. Intense pulsed lightcan be an effective monotherapy or combination treatment for rosacea. Angermeier reported 75% to 100% clearance with 4 IPL sessions with minimal side effects in 200 patients with rosacea, primary telangiectasia, facial hemangiomas, and port wine stains.[20] **Fig. 1** demonstrates a male with rosacea who underwent several treatments to decrease the overall redness to his face. Several other studies were able to demonstrate key improvements including a decrease in blood flow, erythema, and reduction in the telangiectatic areas.[21–23] Due to the advanced nature of rhinophyma, IPL is not an effective treatment for this late-stage condition, which is typically more amenable to surgical correction.

IPL has been shown to cause reversible thermal damage to collagen, inducing contraction of collagen fibers, and fiber remodeling.[24] This effect can produce a photorejuvenation appearance likely due to the overall improvement in skin tone and more even complexion. Even though the results of other studies have confirmed that IPL increases skin elasticity, it has not been shown to affect the reduction of wrinkles.[25] Hedelund and colleagues found that IPL treatment improved skin texture and pigmentation but had no impact on wrinkle reduction.[26]

The most common side effects of IPL treatment can include redness, transient hypersensitivity after procedure, and pain. Other more severe side effects can include edema, bullae, hematoma, crusting, hyper/hypopigmentation, leukotrichia, scarring, keloid formation, and infection.[27] Intense pulsed light is usually avoided in Fitzpatrick skin types IVtoVI due to the increased risk of pigmentation complications and skin injury. It is of particular importance in males to use caution when performing an IPL treatment around facial hair. Due to the broad wavelength spectrum, IPL can inadvertently

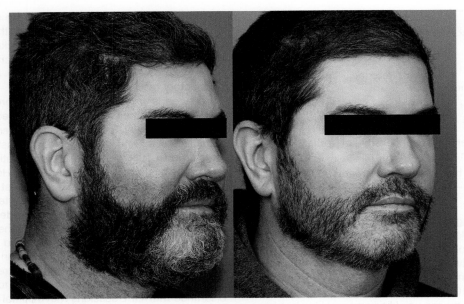

Fig. 1. Demonstrates a male with rosacea who underwent several treatments to decrease the overall redness of his face.

target the melanin in hair follicles, which can cause the hair shaft to heat up. This heat can in turn damage the hair follicle and prevent further growth. This can be particularly problematic when a male does not desire a reduction in his facial hair density. Instructing men to be clean shaven before an IPL treatment and intentionally avoiding the beard distribution can reduce this unwanted side effect from occurring.

Neodymium-doped Yttrium AluminuThe nonablative neodymium-doped yttrium aluminum (Nd:YAG) laser has a wavelength of 1064 nm and has the capability to reach deeper layers of skin tissue than other types of lasers. This laser has been widely used in cosmetic dermatology for the treatment of pigmented and vascular lesions, tattoos, and removal of unwanted hair. The wavelength is absorbed by oxyhemoglobin, melanin, and water and has the capability to penetrate 5 to 6 mm deep into tissues.[28] As was previously discussed, men tend to have a higher concentration of blood vessels than women and are at higher risk for more advanced stages of rosacea. For the treatment of telangiectasias, the Nd:YAG can be very useful as it can heat and cause destruction of the blood vessel wall. The effect is instant as the endothelium and surrounding structures are impacted by a vascular sclerotic process.[29]

Tattoo removal is based on selective photothermolysis, where the ink present in the skin absorbs the energy that is emitted from the laser.[30] The light absorption may also generate a photoacoustic effect that has the ability to destroy the pigment

particle. The ink particles are then broken down by phagocytosis with transfer and elimination via the lymphatic system.[31] Nowadays, the Q-switched and Pico lasers that have shorter pulse durations are desirable for tattoo removal. This can be an effective treatment for those male patients that have tattoos and desire removal.[32,33]

Neodymium-doped yttrium aluminum may also be used for hair removal and is effective for treating dark (brown/black) hair in patients of all skin types.[34] Given the variability of the hair growth cycle, multiple treatments are needed for effective and long-term results. Ismail reported that at a 6-month follow-up after all procedures were completed, patients experienced a 79.4% decrease in hair count.[35] With the effects of androgens on the overall hair density throughout the body, men may be interested in long-term hair removal options in certain regions of the body that they may consider undesirable (back, neck, etc.).

The longer wavelength of the Nd:YAG allows for less melanin absorption. Thus, it is suitable for treating a large range of Fitzpatrick skin types with a markedly decreased risk of dyspigmentation issues at the treated site. Side effects are usually minor and may include pain during treatment, redness, swelling, and bruising. As with many light-based energy devices, effective cooling is essential to avoid any complications associated with overheating the skin such as blisters or superficial injury to the epidermis that can lead to dyspigmentation concerns.

Radiofrequency

Radiofrequency (RF) technology has emerged as an effective minimally invasive treatment for rejuvenation of the skin, particularly on the face and neck. Radiofrequency technology uses electromagnetic waves that cause local hyperthermia by converting electrical energy into intracellular heat following absorption by individual skin structures. The thermal energy that is created incites focal tissue coagulation and a subsequent tissue-repair response. This promotes connective-tissue remodeling and the formation of new collagen, resulting in improved skin elasticity and tissue contraction. The improvement of tension and density of the skin result from contraction of the "old" collagen and stimulation of fibroblasts to produce new fibers.[36] This treatment is safe for all skin types, as it does not cause damage to the melanocytes, if used as indicated in the dermal level, and below.[37] Numerous studies have demonstrated the effects that RF has at the molecular and histopathologic level. These include the upregulation of growth factors, cytokines, and thickening of the papillary dermis, all of which contribute to a reduction in facial rhytids and overall skin tightening.[38–41]

There are 2 main types of RF technology that are used to treat the most common aging skin concerns. Monopolar and bipolar RF are 2 different techniques used to deliver this energy for various purposes, such as skin tightening, fat reduction, and tissue rejuvenation. These techniques differ in how the RF energy is applied and the potential depth of penetration. In monopolar RF, a single electrode is used to deliver the energy to the treatment area. Monopolar RF is often used for procedures that require deeper tissue penetration, such as body contouring and muscle toning. It can also be used for skin tightening, but the depth of penetration can make it less precise for superficial treatments. Bipolar RF utilizes 2 electrodes placed in close proximity to one another on or beneath the skin. The RF energy flows directly between these 2 electrodes, creating a focused field of energy in the tissue between them. Bipolar RF is typically employed for treatments focused on the superficial layers of the skin, including facial rejuvenation, wrinkle reduction, and cellulite reduction. The shallower penetration allows for more controlled and localized heating. This is the most common form of RF energy used for the head and neck and includes microneedling and other minimally invasive devices to heat the dermis.

The periorbital region can be one of the first signs of aging that an individual may notice on his face. Given the dynamic nature of this area, neuromodulators are frequently used as a first-line treatment to manage fine lines and deeper rhytids. Despite the relaxation of the dynamic movement from a neuromodulator, there may still be persistent concerns regarding the overall texture and appearance. Microneedling RF has shown promise in treating this region of the face. Several studies have demonstrated clinical improvement to the static wrinkles in the infraorbital and surrounding area.[42,43] Results tend to be progressive and more noticeable when delivered in a series of 3 treatment sessions on average. In the periorbital region, microneedling RF is reserved mostly for the infraorbital and lateral periorbital region. Monopolar RF has been used to treat the upper eyelid. Biesman and colleagues reported upper eyelid tightening and reduction of hooding in greater than 85% of subjects in a multicenter trial of 72 patients. This non-invasive eyelid treatment can be a reasonable alternative for a male that is not quite ready for surgery but looking for some level of tightening to the upper eyelid. The downtime associated with this is quite minimal. Similar to previous treatments, recommending in a series of 3 is frequently going to yield superior results.

The desire to improve the jawline and contour of the neck continues to increase amongst males.[1] Having a well-balanced and defined jawline is a hallmark of beauty, enhancing the masculine and youthful features on a male face. In recent years, RF technology has been widely applied to many areas of the body for skin tightening and soft-tissue contraction. Several studies have demonstrated acceptable contraction of the underlying tissues on the body, as well as the jawline, submental, and lower lid laxity.[44,45] To improve the contour of the submental area and lateral jawline, RF has been combined with liposuction to produce satisfactory results (**Fig. 2**).[46] This combination becomes particularly important when there is an appreciable amount of submental and lateral subcutaneous fat that is contributing to the fullness in the neck. The addition of RF can complement the reduction of fat by contracting the superficial skin envelope. If any amount of laxity is noted in the consultation, the usage of RF can optimize outcomes, especially in males with a thicker soft-tissue envelope looking to maximize contraction. Potential complications that can arise with this technology include thermal injury, paresis of the marginal mandibular branch of the facial nerve, and transient or permanent hair loss. The issue of hair loss is crucial to discuss with male patients, particularly those that favor some form of a beard, as this can be distressing if they are not informed of possibility of this outcome before the procedure.

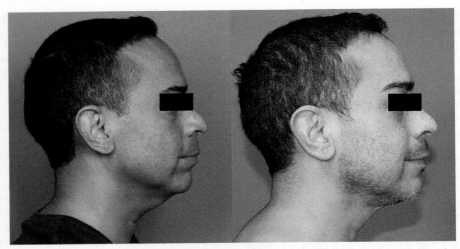

Fig. 2. Demonstrates radiofrequency combined with liposuction to improve the contour of the submental area and lateral jawline.

Ablative Laser Resurfacing

Laser skin resurfacing has become a gold standard option for rejuvenation of the facial skin's texture, tone, and elasticity. For many years, carbon dioxide (CO_2) lasers (wavelength 10,600 nm) were the only lasers available for laser skin rejuvenation. Today other options are available, including the solid-state erbium-doped yttrium aluminum garnet (Er:YAG, 2940 nm). When the Er:YAG laser is applied, it is absorbed by water in the epidermis and papillary dermis. The vaporization of the epidermis leads to the dermal appendages resurfacing the skin in order to heal. The thermal injury in the dermis stimulates collagen production, improving the appearance of photodamaged skin and a reduction in rhytids.[47] The vaporized water acts as a heat sink and decreases the overall amount of thermal injury sustained by the surrounding tissues. This stands in contrast to the CO_2 laser that generates more heat and causes a greater coagulation of small blood vessels in the dermis. Because of this fact, there is typically less bleeding when a large surface is ablated. The chromophore for the CO_2 laser at the 10,600 nm wavelength is intracellular water. A meta-analysis comparing the overall efficacy of CO_2 to Er:YAG showed that the 2 devices do not differ largely in terms of efficacy.[48] Despite there being 2 separate energy-based modalities in the resurfacing category, for the purpose of this article they will be described together as a resurfacing treatment given their similarities in achieving satisfactory results.

Acne scarring is a common consequence of acne. This frequently results from scarring and

reorganizing of the collagen fibers and subcutaneous fat during inflammatory acne vulgaris. The literature suggests more severe inflammation can lead to an increased severity of scarring.[49] This can be emotionally and psychologically distressing, leading to poor self-esteem and reduced daily activities and social interactions. Acne scars can be classified into 3 subtypes: ice-pick scar, rolling scar, and boxcar scar depending on their width, depth, and overall architecture. There are many treatment modalities available that can improve atrophic acne scars. These include chemical peels, dermabrasion, punch grafting, dermal fillers, and ablative and non-ablative lasers. Many of these treatments are operator dependent and as a result can be variable on their efficacies and long-term improvements.[50] It has been shown that adolescent males have a high prevalence of acne scars, some of which are related to their relative socio-economic status and education level. The severity tends to be worse in males as well, possibly related to males having a longer duration of acne, and delaying their treatment. Fractional laser resurfacing is more effective than non-ablative resurfacing for treating acne scars.[51] Some studies were able to show considerable improvement in the appearance of rolling and superficial box acne scars.[52,53] A single treatment for acne scars is not always feasible for this type of scarring, as this tends to be a multimodality and continuous process. Multiple treatments may frequently need to be recommended in order to achieve satisfactory results due to the complex and stubborn nature of acne scars.

In contrast to acne scars, successful treatment of photoaging and rhytids can be achieved in a single treatment depending on the settings used. In contrast to chemical peels and dermabrasion, these devices allow for more precise control over the depth and extent of the thermal damage. The molecular alterations that a CO_2 laser can induce has been demonstrated by Orringer and colleagues They were able to show collagen type I and type III peaking at 7.5 and 8.9 times baseline levels 21 days after treatment to the skin on the forearms.[54] Some of the other benefits of resurfacing can include softening or disappearance of mild-to-moderate rhytids, improved skin texture and tone, decreased pore size, and a reduction in skin laxity. While the downtime is longer than other energy-based treatments, a single treatment can create the most impactful changes to the skin and surrounding tissues and may be more attractive to males. Girdwichai and colleagues evaluated the behaviors and attitudes toward cosmetic treatments among men. Not surprisingly, both sexes preferred gradual improvement with no downtime over complete resolution with 1 treatment and a long recovery period. However, more men preferred the 1 treatment with a longer recovery time option than women did. Additionally, in answer to the question, "Are you willing to go through laser treatment if your dermatologist suggests that it would offer a better outcome?", most men (75.8%) indicated they would undergo laser treatment.[55] This likely explains why males find ablative laser resurfacing an attractive procedure to target many of their skin concerns. Of particular importance is reviewing the post-procedure skincare when choosing a resurfacing modality for a male patient. It has been established that men are less likely than women to apply sunscreen.[56] In order to reduce side effects and complications, a detailed review of care is essential for this population.

SUMMARY

Interest among the minimally invasive facial rejuvenation market has grown amongst the male population in recent years. The desire to remain competitive in the workplace and other social avenues is the likely culprit for this increased interest. Various minimally invasive modalities have been reviewed in this article that can address many of the skin concerns that men are seeking to improve. It is important to set appropriate expectations and understand the motivations for each male patient, as this will ultimately increase the likelihood of a successful cosmetic outcome. This is especially important with minimally invasive treatment options because these devices do not deliver the same results as a surgical option.

CLINICS CARE POINTS

- Male skin produces more sebaceous, eccrine, and apocrine secretions than female skin due to higher levels of testosterone, which can lead to increased sebum production.

- A dose-response relationship between wrinkling and smoking has been identified in addition to an increased incidence of facial elastosis and telangiectasia formation among men.

- Due to the broad wavelength spectrum, IPL can inadvertently target the melanin in hair follicles, causing damage and preventing further growth. This can be particularly problematic when a male does not desire a reduction in his facial hair density.

- Radiofrequency technology can be used as a reasonable alternative for a male that is not quite ready for surgery but looking to address laxity in regions such as the eyelids and jawline.

DISCLOSURE

The author has nothing to disclose.

REFERENCES

1. 2020 Plastic surgery statistics report, *Plastic Surgery*, 2020. Available at: https://www.plasticsurgery.org/documents/News/Statistics/2020/plastic-surgery-statistics-full-report-2020.pdf.
2. Rieder EA, Euphemia WM, Brauer JA. Men and cosmetics: social and psychological trends of an emerging demographic. J Drugs Dermatol JDD 2015;14(9):1023–6.
3. Jagdeo J, Keaney T, Narurkar V, et al. Facial treatment preferences among aesthetically oriented men. Dermatol Surg 2016;42(10):1155–63.
4. Cohen BE, Bashey S, Wysong A. Literature review of cosmetic procedures in men: approaches and techniques are gender specific. Am J Clin Dermatol 2017;18(1):87–96.
5. Luebberding S, Krueger N, Kerscher M. Skin physiology in men and women: in vivo evaluation of 300 people including TEWL, SC hydration, sebum content and skin surface pH. Int J Cosmet Sci 2013;35(5):477–83.
6. Luebberding S, Krueger N, Kerscher M. Mechanical properties of human skin in vivo: a comparative evaluation in 300 men and women. Skin Res Technol 2014;20(2):127–35.
7. Shuster S, Black MM, McVitie E. The influence of age and sex on skin thickness, skin collagen and density. Br J Dermatol 1975;93(6):639–43.

8. Oblong JE. Comparison of the impact of environmental stress on male and female skin. Br J Dermatol 2012;166(Suppl 2):41–4.

9. Vanoosthuyze K, Zupkosky PJ, Buckley K. Survey of practicing dermatologists on the prevalence of sensitive skin in men. Int J Cosmet Sci 2013;35(4):388–93.

10. Hillebrand GG, Liang Z, Yan X, et al. New wrinkles on wrinkling: an 8-year longitudinal study on the progression of expression lines into persistent wrinkles. Br J Dermatol 2010;162(6):1233–41.

11. Luebberding S, Nils K, Martina K. Quantification of age-related facial wrinkles in men and women using a three-dimensional fringe projection method and validated assessment scales. Dermatol Surg 2014;40(1):22–32.

12. Kane MAC, Derek J, Xiaofang L, et al. Heterogeneity of crow's feet line patterns in clinical trial subjects. Dermatol Surg 2015;41(4):447–56.

13. Pinkhasov RM, Wong J, Kashanian J, et al. Are men shortchanged on health? perspective on health care utilization and health risk behavior in men and women in the United States. Int J Clin Pract 2010;64(4):475–87.

14. GBD 2019 Tobacco Collaborators. Spatial, temporal, and demographic patterns in prevalence of smoking tobacco use and attributable disease burden in 204 countries and territories, 1990-2019: a systematic analysis from the global burden of disease study 2019. Lancet (London, England) 2021;397(10292):2337–60.

15. Kennedy C, Maarten TB, Bajdik CD, et al. Bouwes bavinck, and leiden skin cancer study. "effect of smoking and sun on the aging skin.". J Invest Dermatol 2003;120(4):548–54.

16. Falk M, Ashild F, Tomas F. Sun exposure habits and health risk-related behaviours among individuals with previous history of skin cancer. Anticancer Res 2013;33(2):631–8.

17. Beach Holiday Sunburn. The Sunscreen paradox and gender differences - PubMed. Available at: https://pubmed.ncbi.nlm.nih.gov/10431670/. [Accessed 12 October 2023].

18. Weiss RA, Weiss MA, Beasley KL. Rejuvenation of photoaged skin: 5 years results with intense pulsed light of the face, neck, and chest. Dermatol Surg 2002;28(12):1115–9.

19. Scheinfeld N, Berk T. A review of the diagnosis and treatment of rosacea. PGM (Postgrad Med) 2010;122(1):139–43.

20. Angermeier MC. Treatment of facial vascular lesions with intense pulsed light. J Cutan Laser Ther 1999;1(2):95–100.

21. Sadick NS, Weiss R. Intense pulsed-light photorejuvenation. Semin Cutan Med Surg 2002;21(4):280–7.

22. Taub AF. Treatment of rosacea with intense pulsed light. J Drugs Dermatol JDD 2003;2(3):254–9.

23. Schroeter CA, Haaf-von Below S, Neumann HAM. Effective treatment of rosacea using intense pulsed light systems. Dermatol Surg 2005;31(10):1285–9.

24. Patriota RC, Consuelo Junqueira R, Luiz Carlos C. Intense pulsed light in photoaging: a clinical, histopathological and immunohistochemical evaluation. An Bras Dermatol 2011;86(6):1129–33.

25. Shin JW, Lee DH, Choi SY, et al. Objective and non-invasive evaluation of photorejuvenation effect with intense pulsed light treatment in asian skin. J Eur Acad Dermatol Venereol: JEADV 2011;25(5):516–22.

26. Hedelund L, Eva D, Peter B, et al. Skin rejuvenation using intense pulsed light: a randomized controlled split-face trial with blinded response evaluation. Arch Dermatol 2006;142(8):985–90.

27. Radmanesh M, Mohsen A, Arash A, et al. Burning, paradoxical hypertrichosis, leukotrichia and folliculitis are four major complications of intense pulsed light hair removal therapy. J Dermatol Treat 2008;19(6):360–3.

28. Cannarozzo G, Francesca N, Mario S, et al. Q-switched Nd:YAG laser for cosmetic tattoo removal. Dermatol Ther 2019;32(5):e13042.

29. Prieto V, Peter Z, Neil S, et al. Comparison of a Combination Diode Laser and Radiofrequency Device (Polaris) and a Long-Pulsed 1064-Nm Nd:YAG Laser (Lyra) on Leg Telangiectases. Histologic and Immunohistochemical Analysis. J Cosmet Laser Ther 2006;8(4):191–5.

30. Naga LI, Alster TS. Laser tattoo removal: an update. Am J Clin Dermatol 2017;18(1):59–65.

31. Kurniadi I, Farida T, Asnawi M, et al. Laser tattoo removal: fundamental principles and practical approach. Dermatol Ther 2021;34(1):e14418.

32. Qu Y, Wang L, Zhou P, et al. Efficient picosecond laser for tattoo removal in rat models. Med Sci Monit 2020;26:e924583.

33. Elghblawi E. Tattoo removal 'the artistic state of the art.' tattoo on forehead, nose, and chin: successful removal with modified R20 technique using low-fluence Q-switched Nd YAG laser: a case report. J Cosmet Dermatol 2020;19(11):2919–21.

34. Littler CM. Hair removal using an Nd:YAG laser system. Dermatol Clin 1999;17(2):401–30.

35. Ismail SA. Long-Pulsed Nd:YAG laser vs. intense pulsed light for hair removal in dark skin: a randomized controlled trial. Br J Dermatol 2012;166(2):317–21.

36. Hantash BM, Bradley R, Berkowitz R, et al. Pilot clinical study of a novel minimally invasive bipolar microneedle radiofrequency device. Laser Surg Med 2009;41(2):87–95.

37. Battle E, Sally B. Clinical evaluation of safety and efficacy of fractional radiofrequency facial treatment of skin type VI patients. J Drugs Dermatol JDD 2018;17(11):1169–72.

38. El-Domyati M, Tarek S, El-Ammawi WM, et al. Expression of transforming growth factor-β after different non-invasive facial rejuvenation modalities. Int J Dermatol 2015;54(4):396–404.

39. Wakade DV, Nayak CS, Bhatt KD. A study comparing the efficacy of monopolar radiofrequency and glycolic acid peels in facial rejuvenation of aging skin using histopathology and ultrabiomicroscopic sonography (UBM) - an evidence based study. Acta Med 2016;59(1):14–7.

40. Montesi G, Calvieri S, Alberto B, et al. Bipolar radiofrequency in the treatment of dermatologic imperfections: clinicopathological and immunohistochemical aspects. J Drugs Dermatol JDD 2007;6(9):890–6.

41. Tanaka Y, Tsunemi Y, Kawashima M, et al. Treatment of skin laxity using multisource, phase-controlled radiofrequency in asians: visualized 3-dimensional skin tightening results and increase in elastin density shown through histologic investigation. Dermatol Surg 2014;40(7):756–62.

42. Kwon SH, Ji-Young C, Young Ahn G, Woo Sun J, et al. The efficacy and safety of microneedle monopolar radiofrequency for the treatment of periorbital wrinkles. J Dermatol Treat 2021;32(4):460–4.

43. Kim KE, Jong Heon P, Tae Woong S, Il-Hwan K, Hwa Jung R. Periorbital skin rejuvenation of asian skin using microneedle fractional radiofrequency. Ann Dermatol 2023;35(5):360–6.

44. Paul M, Blugerman G, Kreindel M, et al. Three-dimensional radiofrequency tissue tightening: a -proposed mechanism and applications for body contouring. Aesthetic Plast Surg 2011;35(1):87–95.

45. Turer DM, James IB, DiBernardo BE. Temperature-controlled monopolar radiofrequency in the treatment of submental skin laxity: a prospective study. Aesthetic Surg J 2021;41(11):NP1647–56.

46. Zhu J, Tianyi L, Yiqun Z, et al. The application of subcutaneous radiofrequency after liposuction for the lower face and neck contouring under local anesthesia. J Craniofac Surg 2023;34(2):616–9.

47. Riggs K, Matthew K, Tatyana R, et al. Ablative laser resurfacing: high-energy pulsed carbon dioxide and erbium:yttrium-aluminum-garnet. Clin Dermatol 2007; 25(5):462–73.

48. Husein-ElAhmed H, Martin S. Comparative appraisal with meta-analysis of erbium vs. CO2 lasers for atrophic acne scars. Journal Der Deutschen Dermatologischen Gesellschaft 2021;19(11):1559–68.

49. Goodman GJ, Baron JA. Postacne scarring–a quantitative global scarring grading system. J Cosmet Dermatol 2006;5(1):48–52.

50. Fife D. Practical evaluation and management of atrophic acne scars: tips for the general dermatologist. Journal of Clinical and Aesthetic Dermatology 2011;4(8):50–7.

51. Alexiades-Armenakas MR, Dover JS, et al. The spectrum of laser skin resurfacing: nonablative, fractional, and ablative laser resurfacing. J Am Acad Dermatol 2008;58(5):719–37. quiz 738–40.

52. Nirmal B, Pai SB, Handattu S, et al. Efficacy and safety of erbium-doped yttrium aluminium garnet fractional resurfacing laser for treatment of facial acne scars. Indian J Dermatol, Venereol Leprol 2013;79(2):193–8.

53. Schweiger ES, Lauren S. Focal acne scar treatment (FAST), a new approach to atrophic acne scars: a case series. J Drugs Dermatol JDD 2013;12(10): 1163–7.

54. Orringer JS, Sewon Kang TM, Hamilton T, et al. Connective tissue remodeling induced by carbon dioxide laser resurfacing of photodamaged human skin. Arch Dermatol 2004;140(11):1326–32.

55. Girdwichai N, Kumutnart C, Vasanop V. Behaviors and attitudes toward cosmetic treatments among men. Journal of Clinical and Aesthetic Dermatology 2018;11(3):42–8.

56. Roberts CA, Goldstein EK, Karina Paci J, et al. Men's attitudes and behaviors about skincare and sunscreen use behaviors. J Drugs Dermatol JDD 2021;20(1):88–93.

Moving?

Make sure your subscription moves with you!

To notify us of your new address, find your **Clinics Account Number** (located on your mailing label above your name), and contact customer service at:

Email: journalscustomerservice-usa@elsevier.com

800-654-2452 (subscribers in the U.S. & Canada)
314-447-8871 (subscribers outside of the U.S. & Canada)

Fax number: 314-447-8029

Elsevier Health Sciences Division
Subscription Customer Service
3251 Riverport Lane
Maryland Heights, MO 63043

*To ensure uninterrupted delivery of your subscription, please notify us at least 4 weeks in advance of move.

Printed and bound by CPI Group (UK) Ltd, Croydon, CR0 4YY

08/05/2025

01864748-0015